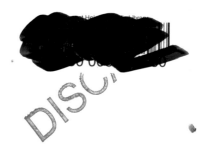

THE WONDER *of the* HUMAN HAND

A JOHNS HOPKINS PRESS HEALTH BOOK

THE WONDER

of the

HUMAN HAND

◆

*Care and Repair of the Body's
Most Marvelous Instrument*

EDITED BY E. F. SHAW WILGIS, M.D.

With Fourteen Experts from the
Renowned Curtis National Hand Center

Johns Hopkins University Press
Baltimore

© 2014 Johns Hopkins University Press
All rights reserved. Published 2014
Printed in the United States of America on acid-free paper
9 8 7 6 5 4 3 2 1

Johns Hopkins University Press
2715 North Charles Street
Baltimore, Maryland 21218-4363
www.press.jhu.edu

Library of Congress Cataloging-in-Publication Data

The wonder of the human hand : care and repair of the body's most marvelous instrument / edited by E. F. Shaw Wilgis, M.D.
   pages cm — (A Johns Hopkins Press health book)
  "With fourteen experts from the renowned Curtis National Hand Center"
  Includes index.
   ISBN 978-1-4214-1547-5 (hardcover : alk. paper) — ISBN 1-4214-1547-X (hardcover : alk. paper) — ISBN 978-1-4214-1548-2 (pbk. : alk. paper) — ISBN 1-4214-1548-8 (pbk. : alk. paper) — ISBN 978-1-4214-1549-9 (electronic) — ISBN 1-4214-1549-6 (electronic) 1. Hand—Physiology—Popular works. 2. Hand—Anatomy—Popular works. 3. Hand—Movements—Popular works. I. Wilgis, E. F. Shaw, editor.
   QP334.W52 2014
   611'.737—dc23   2014006750

A catalog record for this book is available from the British Library.

Special discounts are available for bulk purchases of this book. For more information, please contact Special Sales at 410-516-6936 or specialsales@press.jhu.edu.

Johns Hopkins University Press uses environmentally friendly book materials, including recycled text paper that is composed of at least 30 percent post-consumer waste, whenever possible.

CONTENTS

◆

WORK, PLAY, LOVE

◆

The Marvel of the Human Hand

E. F. Shaw Wilgis, M.D.

> *We have hands; we can stand on them if we want to. That's our*
> *privilege. That's the joy of a mortal body. And that's why God*
> *needs us. Because God loves to feel things through our hands.*
> —Elizabeth Gilbert

As a person who has spent his professional life immersed in the study and practice of medical science, I would like to cite the hand as the anatomy of human progress.

Our hands interact with the environment in ways that are more sophisticated, more varied, and literally more productive than any other part of the body. As the instrument that manifests so much of what the brain is capable of imagining, the hand has been on the front line of history as we have reached, grasped, pinched, and pulled our way to a kinder, safer, more enlightened world. Since the beginning of the species, our progress has been inextricably tied to the marvelous capabilities of our hands.

It is with our hands that we first recorded our immediate environment—offering insight for thousands of later generations—by painting sprawling scenes of humans and animals and daily life on the walls of caves. Our hands did the work when we pushed rocks into place at Stonehenge and thousands of other sites to help us follow what must have been our earliest inkling of the recurring annual seasons. When we carved the Sanskrit of Persia or the hieroglyphics of Egypt, our hands began the written record of our lives. Pens, ink, paper—items conceived by our minds—could not have been fabricated without our hands, nor employed to continually advance human society.

Our hands have played a starring role in helping us meet our most basic needs—food, shelter, clothing. Think about it: the ingenuity of teasing and spinning strands of thread from balls of raw cotton plucked from prickly bolls is a testament to the mind, no doubt. But it is the fine dexterity of the hand that turned a vision into a fiber, and then a woven cloth. And when circumstance allowed a respite from the activities of survival, the hand hammered gold into pieces of adornment, polished carved hunks of marble into works of art, and built musical instruments. From rote, mundane activities to our most sublime achievements as humans, the hand has helped us progress toward a better world and a deeper understanding of our place in it.

Across all cultures and down the millennia of history, our recognition of the significance of the hand is consistently expressed in two universal and exclusively human endeavors: religion and art. In Buddhism, for example, 10 specific hand gestures represent the religion's core moral principles. Called *mudras*, they are instantly recognizable to followers of the faith, and are regularly depicted in Buddhist art (sculptures, paintings) and written chronicles. The mudras, as translated from Sanskrit, are:

- *fearlessness* (formed by an open right palm facing outward at chest level or slightly higher)
- *meditation* (the hands are placed together loosely in the lap with one hand cupping the other, tips of the thumbs touching)
- *greeting and adoration* (palms and fingers of both hands are pressed together flat, held at heart or forehead level)
- *truthfulness* (the left hand is held on the lap, palm up, and the right hand points down to the earth)
- *compassion and sincerity* (usually the left hand, held palm up, fingers and thumb in a relaxed, natural position)

- *expelling evil* (right hand, held palm out at shoulder level, with middle and third fingers bent toward palm while index and small fingers are raised, thumb touching tip of middle finger)
- *confidence / connection with divine energy* (hands are placed flat with palms pressed against middle of chest, crossed, right over left)
- *teaching* (right hand, facing palm out at chest level, the thumb and index finger forming a circle while other fingers are in a relaxed raised position)
- *continuous energy of the cosmic order* (hands are placed at heart level with thumbs and index fingers forming circles, right palm faces out and left palm faces the heart)
- *supreme enlightenment* (both hands placed at the center of the chest, index fingers touching and pointing upward, the other fingers intertwined)

Whatever your faith may be, I encourage you to pause here and make each of these hand positions, reading aloud the word that defines it. I believe you will feel the powerful mind-body connection at work in each one, thanks to the sensitivity of your hands.

In Buddhism, the right hand represents physical work and male traits; the left hand represents wisdom and female traits (or what many cultures since have referred to as "female intuition"). Mudras that call for contact between the right and left hands, then, represent a union of male and female aspects. The picture created by any of the gestures— with one or both hands—is, indeed, worth a thousand words.

As Buddhism spread from India into Nepal, Tibet, China, Thailand, Cambodia, and Japan, the principles represented by the hand gestures translated across multiple languages. The use of the hands as symbols in other religions has been a similar benefit; while spoken languages can block understanding, visual messages created by the hand can be understood anywhere.

In Islamic religious tradition, the hand of the Prophet Muhammad's daughter, Fatima, is viewed as a symbol of patience, faith, loyalty, and protection against difficulties. For centuries, amulets portraying the Hand of Fatima have been fabricated to be displayed or worn for protection, blessing, power, and strength for oneself or one's household. This stylized representation of the hand made its way across North Africa and the Middle East from Islam to Judaism. The symbol of the hand appears in early Jewish manuscripts and is closely connected to letters and words referring to God.

In Hinduism, the oldest religion, the five fingers in the hand represent the five elements of nature and the body's five energy centers (chakra), and representations of the hand are an important symbol in Hindu art as well as in its written and oral history. Amulets and jewelry of the sacred symbol called *Humsa Hand* (the Indian version of the Hand of Fatima) are extremely popular across all socioeconomic groups.

In Christian religious traditions the hand has always been used as a formal expression of faith, blessing, prayer, and praise. Many of the uses of the hand in Christianity mirror those of much earlier religions; the Buddhist mudra for *supreme enlightenment* is the same hand position most Christians use when praying. In the Catholic Church, the hand is used prominently in every ceremony, beginning with baptism. In addition to cupping water in his hand to pour it gently on the infant's head, the priest uses his thumb to trace the sign of the cross (representing the Holy Trinity and dedication to the teachings of the Church) on the baby's forehead.

Over the centuries, art has been an important means of communication for religions, particularly with an illiterate public. Medieval renderings of biblical stories featured the hand in various stylized poses; at a glance, the viewer understood an important moral message. European religious fine art reached a pinnacle during the Renaissance, when a wealthy Roman Catholic Church commissioned works that are still admired today. In this way, the paintings of Fra Angelico, Antonio da Correggio, Leonardo da Vinci, and Michelangelo spoke to the masses on behalf of the Church.

One of the most famous artistic renderings of the hand can be found in Michelangelo's painting *The Creation of Adam*. Part of an enormous fresco he painted in the Sistine Chapel, the detail of the hand of God reaching toward the hand of Adam is one of the most reproduced pieces of art in the world. Even now, 500 years after it was painted, this work enthralls us—no matter what our religious beliefs may be. As a physician dedicated to the care of the hand, I find this painting enormously moving. In it, we see God reaching to touch Adam's hand—not his forehead, or shoulder, or breastbone. Moreover, God is reaching his hand (his index finger, to be precise) to Adam's; we do not find God leaning in to bestow a kiss on the top of Adam's head to infuse him with life. When God uses his outstretched hand to transmit life through Adam's fingers, the symbolic power and marvel of the interaction is there for all to see. It is as if God is saying, "Use your hands wisely; they are your connection to me."

The importance of the hand in art has not been limited to religious works. In secular paintings, from ancient times to the present, the hand conveys information about the person's wealth, social status, and occupation. Rings, long fingers, fine skin, and tidy nails traditionally indicated a person of wealth and education. When a well-to-do gentleman in the eighteenth century commissioned his portrait, it was the fashion to show a delicate, slender, pale, unblemished hand (whether his hands actually looked like that or not); to today's eyes, some of these hands appear to be more feminine than masculine, or just plain unbelievable for the person's age. Note this: whatever your taste in art, if you are a collector, keep in mind that the inclusion of the subject's hands greatly increases the monetary value of a portrait!

Undoubtedly you see hands much more frequently in your day-to-day life than you do in art—religious or secular. Without even thinking about it, you make assumptions about a person's occupation based on his hands; the hands of a stonemason do not usually look like the hands of a professor. A person's marital status is announced on the left hand in the form of a wedding band—one of the most universally recognized cultural symbols. In Western societies, we shake hands as a greeting and when we say goodbye, and in business negotiations a handshake can seal a deal.

From a purely physiological point of view, the hand is an intricately engineered device of 27 bones, 24 muscles, and 32 joints that, when working in concert, allow us to work and to express emotion. Because it is able to sense and return to the brain information not perceived by other body senses, the hand can also help us see, hear, and speak. You could say, "What Watson was to Sherlock Holmes, the hand is to the brain."

As a physician, I chose to specialize in the care of the hand because I find it to be inextricably tied to the human experience, perhaps more so than any other physical aspect with the exception of the brain. Its intricacies captivated me in medical school and its expression of the most sophisticated workings of the brain continues to impress me. Throughout history, the astounding contributions the hand has made possible—the printing press and the advance of literacy; microscopes and the advance of science; sextants and the advance of navigation; the slide-rule and the advance of engineering—has in countless ways made life better.

To me, the beauty and function of the human hand are inseparable from the expression of our humanity. They have carried forward our efforts to bend the natural world to our liking, to improve our environment, and to find meaning in existence. Let us celebrate their remarkable capabilities and use them wisely.

ACKNOWLEDGMENTS

It takes many hands to produce a book. To acknowledge my collaborators is a pleasure.

My thanks go to all of my colleagues who contributed chapters about the various conditions of the hand. They are all present and past members of The Curtis National Hand Center.

In addition, the professionals at Johns Hopkins University Press have been a tremendous help. From the initial idea of this manuscript as part of the health series, Jacqueline Wehmueller has been instrumental. Margaret Murphy took our rough chapters and polished them from our clinical language to something any layperson could understand. My thanks to her and all the rest of the folks at Johns Hopkins University Press who helped produce our final product.

To the artist Jacqueline Schaffer who so elegantly captured the hand in its various shapes and conditions—a special thanks.

To my staff at The Curtis National Hand Center—Anne Mattson, our medical editor; Norm Dubin who refined many of our photographs; and Lorraine Zellers whose patience and caring attitude made the whole project workable—I am grateful to all of you.

Thank you one and all. It could not have been done without you.

THE WONDER *of the* HUMAN HAND

TOUCHED

◆

Hands + Environment = Life

E. F. Shaw Wilgis, M.D.

The mind has exactly the same power as the hands;
not merely to grasp the world, but to change it.
—Colin Wilson

Dr. Raymond M. Curtis, in his 1971 presidential address to the American Society for Surgery of the Hand, said, "I know of no other part of the human body so intimately associated with human behavior. With our hands, we work, play, love, heal, learn, communicate, express our feelings, and make our contributions to society in the form of art, music, literature, and sport."

We agree.

In this book, my fellow writers and I examine the hand and its place in our physical, mental, and emotional world. Because we are hand surgeons and therapists, we explore how birth defects, disease, and injury can affect the hand's function, and what medical science can do to improve or repair the problem. To illustrate the medical information here, we share with you examples of real people—athletes, musicians, artists, doctors, soldiers, and others—who have faced congenital abnormalities, disease, or traumatic injury to the hand. You will also find stories of individuals who use their hands to see or to hear.

In the end, we hope to give you an appreciation of the physical and cognitive nature of the hand—from its in utero appearance as a mere paddle to its skill wielding a surgical scalpel in sophisticated procedures designed to improve hand function and quality of life.

In the first chapter, you will learn about the amazing anatomy of the hand. Understanding the advantages (and disadvantages) of its form helps you see the potential (and limitations) of its function.

Chapter 2 introduces you to the range of congenital causes of less-than-full function of the hand, beginning with difficulties that can start during fetal development. The hand is formed between 5 and 8 weeks after conception, and during this time a number of problems can occur that lead to some kind of limitation in form or function or both. The chapter also examines the various corrective measures that can be considered in these cases.

Chapter 3 focuses on the demands made on the hands of an athlete and the common injuries that result, as well as how some famous professional athletes have adapted to difficult congenital problems. A review of surgical and nonsurgical treatments for athletic injuries is included as well.

Chapter 4 discusses one of the more common problems of the hand—arthritis. Fortunately, much has been learned about how to treat this potentially crippling disease. In this chapter you will learn about the types of arthritis that can affect the hand and the many therapeutic measures—surgical and nonsurgical—that can be employed to relieve pain, correct deformities, and improve function.

Chapter 5 examines the stresses regularly made to the hands of a musician, and how and when medical attention can help. For the audience, a performance of classical music can seem serene and ethereal; it may be surprising to learn just how demanding the physical toll of professional musicianship can be. Corrective measures, surgical and nonsurgical, are given here, as are suggestions for avoiding injuries and a practice schedule for returning to play after a setback.

Chapter 6 explores how the hand helps the deaf communicate both with one another and with the hearing world. You will learn how American Sign Language was developed, as well as how a hand surgeon can help when a deaf individual has a physical or functional deficiency in his hand.

Chapter 7 is, we hope, both a cautionary and an encouraging tale of hand injuries at home and at work, and how they can and should be treated medically. Make note: even if you work at a computer all day, you are "working" with your hands. You will learn about injury prevention in this chapter as well.

Chapter 8 shows you the toll diabetes can take on hand function. Many people think of diabetes as little more than a "nuisance" disease, requiring monitoring of blood sugar levels. The truth is, diabetes can cause serious problems throughout the body, including the hands. Because diabetes is a disease that has reached epidemic levels, the information in this chapter will be important to many.

Chapter 9 is about the remarkable development of Braille and the use of the fingertips to read. The hand plays an amazing role in helping the blind navigate a seeing world. Sometimes, as you will learn, a hand surgeon can help a blind person "see" better. To a blind person, the sensitivity of her fingertips is as essential as eyes are to a sighted person.

Chapter 10 covers the contracted and spastic effects that some congenital diseases (or damage to the hand from other causes) can result in and what medical science can do to correct or improve them. You will learn, for instance, about Dupuytren contracture, and how this famous malady is depicted in art. Varied spastic conditions that can occur early or late in life, and the measures that can be employed to correct them, are included here, too.

The final chapter, chapter 11, is dedicated to the amazing advances being made in the field of hand surgery, including hand transplantation. Tissue transfer for reconstruction, chemical treatment of spastic problems, muscle and nerve transfer to restore function—a host of sophisticated surgical treatments and the history of their development are discussed. The contents of this chapter are a testament to the continually astounding creativity and perseverance of medical pioneers dedicated to the treatment of the human hand.

The comments of a man who spoke recently during a celebration at The Curtis National Hand Center captured the essence of why my colleagues and I do what we do. Born with an incomplete hand, he recounted his experience of being "liberated to simply live life" thanks to the work of Dr. Curtis. He explained:

In the summer of 1955, Dr. Curtis built—with very little raw material to work with—two small fingers on my left hand. All he had to work with were five small lumps. Only the thumb had any joints and the joint at the base that would allow it to move was almost an inch and a half under the surface. Buried next to the thumb's base, nestled far too close to the thumb to move or grasp even the smallest objects, lay a small index finger.

One of Dr. Curtis's contributions to my life is that I seldom think, much less talk about, my hand. Although being able to tie one's shoes beats not being able to, it's about how, in enabling people to do life's myriad little tasks unselfconsciously and naturally, you liberate them to focus on living life to the fullest, to be known by the quality of their actions, by the goodness in their hearts, by their character and values. You have given them the chance, in the words of the children's poem, "to be the best of whatever you are."

My fellow writers and I, current or former faculty members of The Curtis National Hand Center at MedStar Union Memorial Hospital in Baltimore, Maryland, have devoted our professional lives to the care of the hand. Ours is a book that, we hope, will give you a new understanding of the human hand, from its remarkable anatomy and function to its essential role in the advancement of human society through the ages. Our clinical research, our roles as teachers of orthopedic and plastic surgeons-in-training, and our experience as specialists treating thousands of patients over the years have been gratifying and humbling. Our patients continue to teach and inspire us every day.

We hope you will find our book enlightening and—if you or a loved one has a hand problem—encouraging.

CHAPTER 1

FORM FOLLOWS FUNCTION

◆

The Anatomy of the Hand

Ryan D. Katz, M.D.

There is something poetic about the human hand. The beautiful synergy of its form and function is indeed the "visible part of the brain." This most delicate appendage is able to knead bread dough and perform a heart transplant, throw a baseball and knit a sweater, play the piano, and close a wound with suture. Our hands can hold a piece of charcoal and render a portrait, tap a keyboard and record history, create a scale model of a skyscraper and build that skyscraper.

In the hand, complex coordinated motion is generated by some of the most delicate parts of the body—small articulating bones; a network of tendons; multiple nerves with unique endpoints and functions (some sensory, some motor); diminutive arteries, veins, and muscles; and skin. Pause for a moment: tie your shoelace slowly and deliberately, and watch this poetry in motion. Then, ask yourself how it's possible that you perform such a complicated activity every day—easily, quickly, and without thought. The answer: the amazing human hand.

The stability and shape of your hand arises from the underlying skeleton (see figure 1.1 A). There are 27 bones in each hand: 8 carpal bones, 5 metacarpals, and 14 phalanges.

A

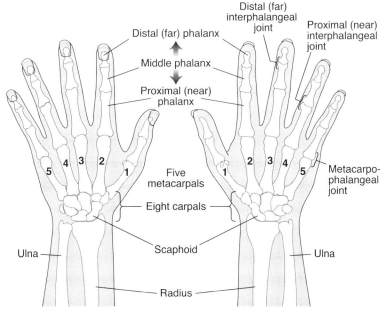

Distal (far) phalanx

Distal (far) interphalangeal joint

Proximal (near) interphalangeal joint

Middle phalanx

Proximal (near) phalanx

5 4 3 2 1

Five metacarpals

1 2 3 4 5

Metacarpo-phalangeal joint

Eight carpals

Scaphoid

Ulna

Ulna

Radius

Bones and joints of left hand
(Back view with forearm)

Bones and joints of left hand
(Palm-side view with forearm)

B

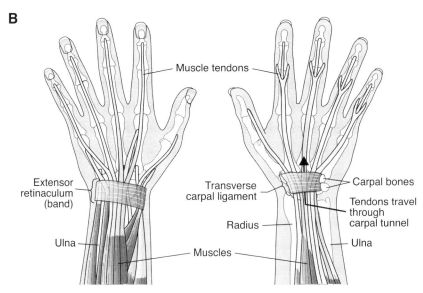

Muscle tendons

Extensor retinaculum (band)

Transverse carpal ligament

Carpal bones

Tendons travel through carpal tunnel

Radius

Ulna

Ulna

Muscles

**Extrinsic extensor muscles
and tendons of left hand**
(Back view with forearm)

**Extrinsic flexor muscles
and tendons of left hand**
(Palm-side view with forearm)

C

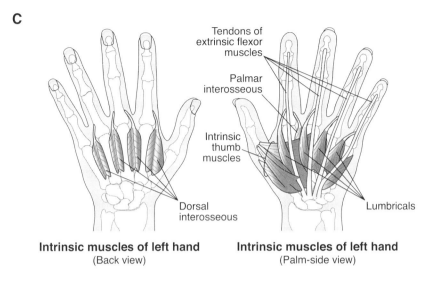

Tendons of
extrinsic flexor
muscles

Palmar
interosseous

Intrinsic
thumb
muscles

Dorsal
interosseous

Lumbricals

Intrinsic muscles of left hand
(Back view)

Intrinsic muscles of left hand
(Palm-side view)

Figure 1.1. (A) Bones and joints of the left hand; (B) extrinsic extensor muscles and tendons of the left hand; (C) intrinsic muscles of the left hand. ILLUSTRATION BY JACQUELINE SCHAFFER

BONES AND JOINTS OF THE HAND

The *carpal bones* serve as a dynamic connection between the long bones of the forearm (*radius* and *ulna*) and the fingers of the hand. Each of the eight carpal bones has a unique shape and makes a singular contribution to wrist motion. The *scaphoid*, a bone with a dugout boat–like appearance that derives its etymology from the Greek word *skaphe* (boat), serves as a link between the two rows of carpal bones. This bone is worthy of mention as it is the most commonly fractured carpal bone. It is almost entirely covered by cartilage and has a tenuous blood supply. Because of the scaphoid's limited blood flow, fractures can be slow to heal or may not heal at all. When a scaphoid fracture does not heal, the bone collapses and the link between the two rows of carpal bones becomes compromised. The result is a progressive degenerative change in the wrist joint, usually accompanied by pain and arthritis.

The five *metacarpal bones* are the long bones of the hand. These bones appear most prominently when the hand is in a fist position. In this pose, the knuckles you see are the "heads" of the metacarpals. The ring and small finger metacarpals have significantly more motion at their bases than do the index and middle fingers. The added mobility at the ring and small finger knuckles gives the hand a more powerful grip, helpful, for example, when using a hammer. Without this extra movement, it would be difficult to grasp small cylindrical objects with force.

The index and middle finger metacarpals, however, do not have this kind of motion at their bases. Boxers and trained professional fighters take advantage of this structural stability and train to "contact" their opponents with the knuckles of their index and middle fingers. Striking a blow with these knuckles allows for a direct transmission of force—from the body to the arm through the hand to the stable metacarpals—into the opponent. By contrast, brawlers or untrained fighters often "contact" their opponents with the more mobile (and therefore less efficient transmitters of force) ring and small finger knuckles, frequently resulting in fractures of one or both fingers. These fractures have come to be called *boxer's fractures*, although the term *brawler's fractures* may be more appropriate because true boxers avoid striking opponents with their small and ring fingers.

The 14 *phalanges* are the bones of the fingers. Each finger has 3 phalanges and the thumb has 2. These small tubular bones articulate with each other and, together with the metacarpals, form the finger joints. The knuckles you see when you make a fist are called the *metacarpophalangeal joints*, and the knuckles you see when you bend your fingers or thumb are the *interphalangeal joints*.

In the fingers, the joint closest to the nail is called the *distal (far) interphalangeal joint*. This joint is often affected by osteoarthritis, the result of "wear and tear" to the cartilage. The next joint is called the *proximal (near) interphalangeal joint*. With an average motion arc of 110 degrees, the proximal interphalangeal joint is the greatest contributor to the finger's range of motion (the total range of motion for a healthy finger is around 270 degrees). Injury to the proximal interphalangeal joint can be quite debilitating, limiting the hand's ability to function fully.

MUSCLES AND TENDONS OF THE HAND

Gross, or big, motions of the hand are a result of the muscles and tendons of the forearm. These muscles are called *extrinsic muscles of the hand* because they originate next to the hand, not within it. Making a tight fist will allow you to see (and feel) the extrinsic *flexor* muscles contracting at their origin by the inside of the elbow. Looking at the back of your forearm while extending your fingers out straight will allow you to see the extrinsic *extensor* muscles working. The extrinsic flexor and extensor muscles travel from the forearm to the fingers via long *tendons* (see figure 1.1 B). The *tendons* are parallel bundles of collagen arranged in a configuration that, like a large steel cable made up of smaller steel cables, has significant strength.

There are two extrinsic flexor tendons for every finger and one extrinsic flexor for the thumb. That means nine flexor tendons must make their way from the forearm to the fingers. They do so by traveling through a tight tunnel at the wrist. This tunnel is called the *carpal tunnel*. The carpal tunnel, which has carpal bones as its "floor" (the back of the hand) and a tight ligament (the transverse carpal ligament) as its "roof" (the palm side of the hand), contains more than just the nine extrinsic flexor tendons; it also contains the median nerve.

NERVES OF THE HAND

The *median nerve* is a large peripheral nerve that travels from the brain all the way to the tips of the fingers (see figure 1.2 A). This nerve provides sensation to the thumb, index finger, middle finger, and half of the ring finger. It also carries a motor branch that innervates the small intrinsic muscles of the thumb. (*Intrinsic muscles* are those whose origin and insertion are within the hand; see figure 1.1 C.) When the median nerve is pinched or compressed, the result is numbness or tingling in the thumb, index finger, and middle finger. If it is pinched severely enough, complete numbness in those digits as well as a wasting away of the intrinsic musculature of the thumb can result. This condition—pressure of the median nerve at the wrist causing numbness and tingling (and, in severe cases, diminishing of the thumb muscle's bulk)—is known as *carpal tunnel syndrome* (see chapter 9).

Carpal tunnel syndrome can be mild, moderate, or severe. Diagnosis is determined through a careful review of the person's history, a physical exam, and, sometimes, electrodiagnostic studies performed by a neurologist. The first line of treatment for mild carpal tunnel syndrome is a wrist splint (worn at night) and oral anti-inflammatory medications. When these treatments are not effective, or if the condition is causing muscle loss in the thumb, surgical treatment is considered. During the surgical procedure, the surgeon releases the "roof" of the carpal tunnel by cutting the transverse carpal ligament, making space for the nine tendons and median nerve to pass through the tunnel without compression.

There are more intrinsic muscles in the hand than just those of the thumb. These include specialized intrinsic muscles to the small finger as well as two groups of intrinsic muscles to the remaining fingers. The intrinsic muscles to the fingers originate either between the metacarpals (called *interossei*) or from the deep extrinsic flexor tendons (called *lumbricals*) The lumbricals are the only muscles in the human body to originate and insert on a tendon. All of these small intrinsic muscles give strength to the hand and assist in fine movements of the fingers. Without these muscles, grasping and manipulating objects is difficult (if not impossible), even when the extrinsic muscles are working properly.

With few exceptions, most of the intrinsic muscles of the hand are activated by the *ulnar nerve*. The ulnar nerve is another large peripheral nerve that travels from the brain to the tips of the fingers. Like the median nerve, the ulnar nerve can be pinched or compressed. Unlike the median nerve, however, compression of the ulnar nerve most often occurs at the elbow, at a place called the *cubital tunnel*. When you hit your "funny bone," what you are really striking is your ulnar nerve at the cubital tunnel. Compression of the ulnar nerve at this point can cause numbness and tingling in the small and ring fingers and, if severe enough, weakness and wasting of the intrinsic hand muscles.

Like carpal tunnel syndrome, ulnar nerve compression is usually treated with the most conservative, least invasive measures first. Wearing a splint that keeps the arm straight during sleep and taking anti-

A

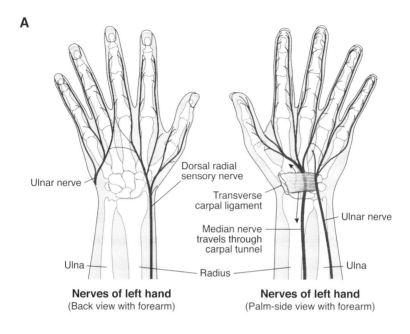

Nerves of left hand
(Back view with forearm)

Ulnar nerve

Dorsal radial
sensory nerve

Transverse
carpal ligament

Median nerve
travels through
carpal tunnel

Ulna

Radius

Nerves of left hand
(Palm-side view with forearm)

Ulnar nerve

Ulna

B

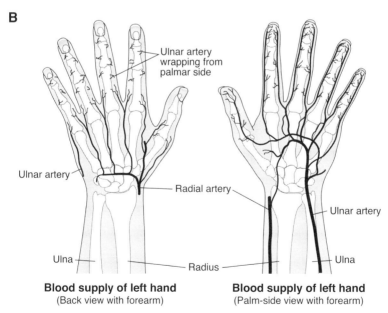

Ulnar artery
wrapping from
palmar side

Ulnar artery

Radial artery

Ulna

Radius

Blood supply of left hand
(Back view with forearm)

Ulnar artery

Ulna

Blood supply of left hand
(Palm-side view with forearm)

Figure 1.2. (A) Nerves of the left hand; (B) blood supply of the left hand. ILLUSTRATION BY JACQUELINE SCHAFFER

inflammatory medications is a good starting point. If the symptoms become severe enough, ulnar nerve compression can be addressed with a surgical procedure to release the nerve. Sometimes, the surgeon will also move the ulnar nerve to a new position to minimize tension on it during flexion. This surgery is called a *transposition*.

Another nerve that travels to the hand is the *radial nerve*. The radial nerve takes a circuitous course, branching from the brachial plexus, traveling along the back of the humerus (under the triceps), then coursing across the front of the arm just above the elbow only to dive to the back again just below the elbow. Before it heads to the back of the forearm, the radial nerve gives off a large sensory branch that travels in a relatively straight fashion down to the wrist. This branch, called the *dorsal radial sensory nerve* (DRSN), lies close to the surface at the wrist and is vulnerable to damage from blunt trauma, laceration, or compression.

Compression of the DRSN at the level of the wrist is called *Wartenberg syndrome*. This syndrome can be treated surgically, by releasing the point of nerve compression, but every effort to manage the condition nonsurgically should be exhausted first. These approaches include removal of all circumferential accessories at the wrist (watch, bracelets, etc.) and the use of oral anti-inflammatory medicine. Surgery carries with it the risk of nerve injury, which is why operative treatment should only be considered after all nonsurgical treatments have failed to provide relief.

In addition to the sensory fibers described above, the radial nerve also carries motor fibers that activate all of the extrinsic extensor muscles on the back of the forearm. Because of the radial nerve's close proximity to the humerus (the arm bone), a humerus fracture can pinch, trap, or injure the radial nerve. When injured, the radial nerve can cause *wrist drop*—the loss of the ability to extend the wrist and fingers. A wrist drop can also occur when a mass (such as a cyst or tumor) presses on the motor branch of the radial nerve in the back of the forearm.

When a person experiences spontaneous wrist drop, an MRI (magnetic resonance imaging) of the forearm is performed to rule out the presence of a cyst or tumor. If the doctor does not expect the nerve to recover, loss of wrist and finger extension can be corrected surgically with *tendon transfers*. This procedure involves taking healthy muscle tendons from elsewhere in the forearm and rerouting them to establish active motion where it has been lost. Tendon transfers can also be used to restore balance to the wrist and fingers when other nerve injuries have affected mobility.

BLOOD SUPPLY TO THE HAND

There are two main arteries to the hand, the *radial artery* and the *ulnar artery*. These two vessels are best appreciated at the wrist. The radial artery is on the thumb side of the wrist and is often felt when taking a person's pulse. Press the tip of your middle finger there now and you'll feel it. The ulnar artery (located on the small finger side of the wrist) is deeper—directly under the stout flexor carpi ulnaris tendon—and therefore somewhat more difficult to feel (see figure 1.2 B).

There is debate among physicians as to which artery is more important to the hand. In a young, otherwise healthy person, the hand can survive on either artery alone. Even in people with coronary artery disease, the hand can survive with just one artery—we know this to be true because the radial artery is sometimes harvested by cardiac surgeons to be used for *coronary artery bypass grafting* (CABG).

That said, hands affected by vascular disease or with anatomic variations cannot tolerate injury to or loss of (by surgical "harvest") either one of these dominant blood vessels. In such situations, the fingers become cool to the touch and the loss of circulation causes pain. If a finger's demand for oxygen cannot be met by the supply delivered by a diseased or injured blood vessel, the finger will not survive. This scenario can be seen in persons with severe vascular disease or autoimmune disorders of the blood vessels. In some cases, a surgeon may be able to help prevent tissue loss by bypassing the diseased blood vessels (*arterial bypass*), performing a *sympathectomy* (which prevents blood vessels from contracting), or by diverting blood from the arterial system to the venous system (*venous arterialization*).

Blood to the fingertips can also be disrupted by an *embolus*, more commonly known as a clot. Think of an embolus as a projectile that originates "upstream" from the fingers. If bacteria have taken up residence on a heart valve, for example, pieces of clot and debris can flick off and travel "downstream" to the hand, getting stuck in one of the small vessels of the wrist or hand. The person experiencing an embolus would feel a sudden onset of pain and coolness in the affected digits. There may also be painful purple lesions on the pads of fingertips and small hemorrhages under nails. Causes of this condition vary; it can be seen in those who abuse intravenous drugs, those with heart valve anomalies, or those with aneurysms of their large vessels. Treatment involves identifying and correcting the problem "upstream" and removing, bypassing, or dissolving the "downstream" obstruction.

SKIN AND SOFT TISSUE

Very specialized skin and soft tissue protect our hands from the environment. The skin on the back of the hand is hair-bearing, loose, and pliable. This laxity allows the fingers to flex without being tethered. The hair-bearing skin on the back of your hand is clearly different from the skin of your palm. The palm skin, called *glabrous* skin, is thick, relatively immobile, and packed with specialized nerve appendages. These appendages allow you to feel pain and to ascertain temperature, light touch, vibration, and position—and seamlessly transmit this information to your brain.

Immediately beneath the palm skin is fat and *palmar fascia*. The palmar fascia is a mat of collagen that has strong attachments to the overlying skin. It can aid in grasping and holding objects in the palm. In some people, this fascia can become thickened and fibrotic. When that happens, the fascia can pull on the skin and fingers and cause subcutaneous nodules, skin pits, and finger contractures. This condition, called *Dupuytren disease* (discussed in detail in chapter 10), appears to have both a genetic and an environmental component, though the specific causes remain unclear. If severe enough, the resulting finger contractures can interfere with everyday activities and make what are usually easy motions, such as placing your hands in your pockets or flat on the top of a table, impossible.

Today, Dupuytren disease can be treated surgically or nonsurgically.

The surgical treatments include *fasciectomy* (removal of the diseased fascia) or *fasciotomy* (cutting into the fascia to release the tethering effect on the finger). Nonsurgical treatments include *needle aponeurotomy* (using a needle to perforate the fascia cords in multiple places, allowing the cords to break) or *collagenase injections* (injecting a chemical that breaks down collagen, allowing the cords to break). Each treatment carries with it risks and benefits best described by the patient's hand surgeon.

THE ANATOMY OF PROGRESS

What first appears as a solid paddle after 30 days of intrauterine existence is formed into a recognizable hand between the fifth and eighth week of gestation, setting the stage for what is perhaps, other than the brain, our most important physical tool. From the underlying bone to its overlying skin, the delicate anatomy and astounding usefulness of the hand command our admiration and awe. Our hands are fine-precision tools and the basis of much of our self-expression. They are, quite simply, the anatomy of human progress.

◆

In the chapters to follow, you will learn about genetic, traumatic, and disease-based affronts to this beautiful tool. You will also learn what medical science can do to restore hand function as fully as possible, as well as how individuals with a hand deficit of one kind or another have still managed to lead remarkable lives.

CHAPTER 2

LESS (OR MORE) THAN A PERFECT 10

◆

Congenital Differences

Michael A. McClinton, M.D.

The birth of a child is a truly magical event, and its anticipation brings great excitement not only to the expectant mother and father but also to the entire family. Before he is even born, the child is deeply loved. Virtually all prospective relatives—grandparents, aunts, uncles, siblings, cousins—begin to imagine how they will nurture, support, guide, and simply adore the baby once he arrives. It is no wonder, then, that the birth of a child with any physical or mental abnormality can be emotionally devastating. Parents grieve for the future they had imagined for the child and mourn the challenges he will face (difficulties that are meaningless to the infant).

Once in every 1,500 births, a child is born with a significant abnormality of the hand and/or arm, what is called a *congenital difference of the upper limb*. The condition can be inherited, and one that is already well-known to the family. Indeed, if it is recognized as a dominant genetic trait, the abnormality may even have been expected. But more than half of the time, the limb anomaly is not an inherited condition and is totally unexpected.

The encouraging news is that many of the more common congenital hand differences can often be addressed with medical intervention. But even when there is not much that can be done to improve the function of the hand or upper limb, many individuals, as you will see in this chapter, still manage not only to live full lives but also to make significant contributions to society—achievements that would be considered remarkable in a completely able-bodied person. I hope you will find their stories inspiring.

THE ONE-ARMED MAJOR LEAGUE BASEBALL PLAYER

In the United States, the best-known athlete with a serious upper limb deficiency was a Major League Baseball pitcher named Jim Abbott (figure 2.1). Jim was born in Flint, Michigan, in 1967, without a right hand. His left limb was normal; more than that, it proved to be a "golden arm." In high school, he played two sports and was a standout pitcher and quarterback. He went on to attend the University of Michigan, where he led his college baseball team to two Big 10 Conference championships. In 1987, he won the James E. Sullivan Award as the top amateur athlete in the United States, the first pitcher ever to win this award. He pitched in the 1988 Summer Olympics, winning the final game and leading the U.S. team to the Gold Medal.

That same year, Abbott was drafted by the California Angels and went on to enjoy a 10-year Major League Baseball career, capped on September 4, 1993, when he pitched a no-hitter for the New York Yankees. Fans marveled at the speed with which he would throw the pitch and immediately transfer the glove from the end of his right arm to his left

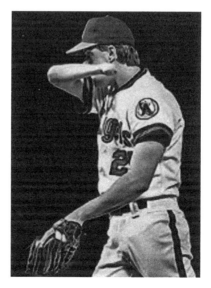

Figure 2.1. Jim Abbott, Major League Baseball player. COURTESY JIM ABBOTT

hand to field any baseballs hit in his direction. Once he had made the catch, he would secure the glove and baseball between his right forearm and torso, slip his left hand out of the glove, and throw the ball to first base. Opposing teams tried to exploit this disadvantage by bunting to him, but the tactic rarely was successful. After retiring from professional baseball, Abbott became a motivational speaker. In 2007, he was elected to the College Baseball Hall of Fame. He is a true inspiration for all, particularly children with a congenital limb difference.

A SURGEON WITHOUT FINGERS

Dr. Liebe Diamond, a well-known pediatric orthopedist, was born with only partial fingers. It was 1931 and hand surgery was not yet a specialty. Her parents, however, took her to a surgeon with a creative mind who gradually addressed her problems; by the time Liebe was a teenager, she had undergone more than 25 surgeries.

From the start, the doctor strongly recommended that Liebe's parents send her to public school so she wouldn't be pampered because of her obvious hand abnormality. As an adult, Dr. Diamond recalled how fortunate she had been in this regard. "I was lucky to have parents who didn't spoil me and made me fend for myself," she said. By the time she was a young woman, she completely accepted her physical differences, thinking, "This is the way you are. This is the way you are going to be." She would tell her friends, "You can either bitch and moan and make everyone around you miserable or accept what is reality and get on with your life."

Dr. Diamond did get on with her life. She graduated from Smith College and went on to the University of Pennsylvania Medical School and a residency program in orthopedic surgery—even though she was missing four fingers on one hand "and the other hand didn't look so great" (figure 2.2). She had a successful career, married, and became a mother and, later, a grandmother. When the piano and French horn were not within her reach because of the fingering issues, she learned to play the trumpet. "I did just about everything I wanted to do . . . I even became a good carpenter!" She always thought it was important

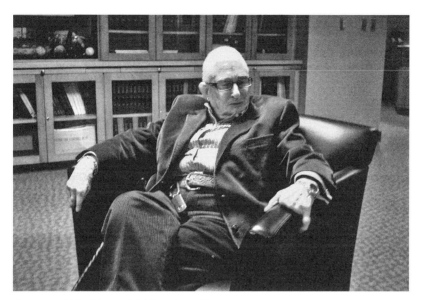

Figure 2.2. Liebe Diamond, M.D., orthopedic surgeon. COURTESY NORMAN H. DUBIN, PH.D.

not to be shy about her hands, and didn't try to hide them from view. During her career as a surgeon (which she managed with custom-made gloves) she specialized in hand and limb deformities in children, an area completely overlooked in the orthopedic community at the time. Eventually, Dr. Diamond gained a national and international reputation for her work.

WHEN THERE IS A PROBLEM: THREE POINTS OF VIEW

A congenital abnormality that causes differences in the appearance and function of the infant's hand affects the parents as well as the child. Their perspectives may differ, as may that of the hand surgeon they consult. Each has a unique point of view worth considering.

The Effect on the Child

Although the parents are deeply affected, albeit indirectly, it is the child who is directly affected by the congenital condition that has caused the abnormal appearance and function of her hand or upper limb. In the words of Richard Smith, a well-known hand surgeon who chaired the Division of Hand Surgery at Massachusetts General Hospital in Boston from 1972 to 1987, "The hand is the only part of the body that is always visible to the patient." Any abnormality, then, is a continuous reminder to the child from at least school age on that she is different from virtually every one of her peers.

Unlike an injury to a "normal" hand, an abnormal hand that is the result of a congenital condition is, for the affected child, a normal hand. Young children typically make the best functional use of their hands, however impaired they may be. Eventually, though, the abnormal hand will become a source of increasing frustration, particularly when the child is unable to participate in the activities of childhood with the ease of peers—or at all. In addition, children with readily apparent hand differences are often the target of mean-spirited comments by other children, which can cause emotional withdrawal and loneliness. One can only imagine how difficult it is during the teen years, when there is such a strong emphasis on appearance and conformity.

The human hand grows quickly, virtually doubling in size between birth and 2 years of age, and then doubling in size again by the end of adolescence. To match the needs of the growing child with a congenital hand abnormality, the hand surgeon's goals include obtaining pinch function between the thumb and index finger by 1 year of age, and completing all or most of the other needed surgical procedures before the child begins first grade. This is the age when the function of the hand becomes even more important to the child's learning experience and is also the time when any hand abnormalities become especially apparent to other children.

The Effect on the Parents and Family

The parents of a child with a significant physical problem that affects appearance or function (or both) often experience a flood of emotions, including guilt and anger. It is imperative that parents take steps to deal with any negative emotions so they can focus on supporting their child with complete attention. It is also important for parents to establish a solid rapport with the child's pediatrician and hand surgeon early on. Many of the decisions that lie ahead require an informed partnership.

"Can you make my child's hand normal?" is usually the first question parents ask the doctor. While the question is straightforward, the answer is not.

When you first meet with the hand surgeon, be sure to bring a notepad and pen and a list of all the questions you hope to have answered. It is important to realize, though, that although many conditions can benefit from hand surgery and therapy, some conditions cannot be improved. Each case is unique. Often, the most important part of the conversation the hand surgeon will have with the parents is explaining that their child's hand will never be completely restored, in either appearance or function. There are usually, however, a variety of good treatment options. Determining the best ones for your child is a decision the hand surgeon will help you make.

Some parents are filled with a sense of great urgency and believe they must make a quick decision about treatment, particularly if surgical reconstruction of their child's hand is an option. Their thinking is, *Let's start now!* Other parents are so overwhelmed by the situation, they find themselves unable to make any decision about the child's treatment, despite multiple consultations with different surgeons.

The fact is, there is almost never a need to rush to surgical treatment, as virtually no congenital hand difference requires urgent treatment. Take your time. The surgeon may suggest that you speak with parents of children who have similar conditions, to learn from their experiences. If this opportunity is offered to you, take it; you will find it tremendously helpful. In addition, the Internet can provide helpful information about congenital hand differences. (You will find a list of organizations that provide help to parents of children with congenital hand abnormalities in the resources section at the end of this book.)

As an orthopedic surgeon specializing in hand and limb deformities in children, Dr. Liebe Diamond saw many abnormal hands. In addition to treating the child, she faced deeply distressed parents who needed reassurance. "You cannot tell on the day a child is born what that child is going to do or become," she would tell them. "You have to be forward-looking and pluck away at the problems and provide the child with the best function." Often, a parent's biggest concern was the appearance of the child's hand. Dr. Diamond, born with significant hand abnormalities, understood that a hand that "worked" was paramount; cosmetic concerns, while important, were secondary. As she noted, "The most invisible hand is the one that functions best."

The Surgeon's Perspective

Well before any surgical procedures are discussed or carried out, let the surgeon play a supportive role; he understands the strain on the family and wants to alleviate it. This may mean that, at first, the surgeon will spend more time communicating with you, the parents, than examining your child. A thorough explanation of the cause of the condition, if known, is a good starting point. Next, a review of all the realistic options for treatment can be discussed. The initial evaluation will involve a history of the pregnancy as well as a genetic history of the family to look for relatives who may be affected by a similar condition.

The physical examination of the child will include the affected limb, an evaluation of the other arm; a review of the shoulder and elbow above the affected hand, and a general survey of the child's musculoskeletal system. The examination may also include photographs of the affected limb or video documentation of the child using her hands and arms. X-rays are often taken, although in the early months of life only some of the bones will be *ossified* (sufficiently hardened) enough to be visible. It is generally impractical to use more sophisticated imaging (CT [computed tomography] scanning or MRI [magnetic resonance imaging]) for an infant or young child because they will not be able to remain still long enough for the study to be completed.

Dr. Adrian Flatt, director of the Division of Hand Surgery at the University of Iowa for more than 20 years beginning in the late 1950s and considered a leader in the description of congenital anomalies, identified the goals of hand surgery for children as follows:

- Ideally, the child should be able to place the hand in space to position it for carrying out activities.
- The hand and wrist should have stable skin coverage with good sensation.

- The hand should be capable of power grasp and precision handling for manipulation of large and small objects.

For children with severe congenital differences, only some of these goals will be achievable. Once the goals of surgery have been identified, the surgeon should provide the parents with as much information as possible about pre-surgical preparation, the procedure itself, and the post-surgical regimen that will need to be followed. Any need for pre-operative splints or casts, the type of pre-operative evaluations that will be required, and anesthesia options based on the child's age and weight will all be discussed. (Virtually all operations for congenital hand differences are carried out under general anesthesia.) In addition, many operations require temporary or permanent pinning of affected joints. Post-operative considerations include the number and location of incisions, the types of sutures (most skin sutures placed in children are the dissolving type), and the type of splinting and casting and length of time they will be needed after the surgical procedure. To ensure a safe procedure, the hand surgeon will generally refer you to a specialist to investigate whether the child has any bleeding or cardiac conditions.

As you can see, there's a lot of information to cover. As a hand surgeon, I find that only the simplest problems can be adequately reviewed with the family in a single visit. Often, two to three visits are needed. Multiple visits also allow you and the child to become comfortable with the surgeon while fully learning about the available options. The hand surgeon's overwhelming obligation is always to make the hand a better functioning unit.

When the child is very young or still a baby, he is not able to participate in the decision-making process. Some parents, because of a desire to include the child's preferences in the choice of treatment options, will opt to postpone decisions about surgery until the child matures. Unfortunately, this delay may deny the child the opportunity to have an improved, better functioning hand. Each case is unique, and the surgeon will be able to advise you of the hazards, if there are any, of holding off on a decision.

DEVELOPMENT OF THE UPPER LIMB

Embryologists have learned a lot about the prenatal development of the hands. The first appearance of what will become the arm and hand (the upper limb) occurs at 25 days after fertilization and is only a protrusion (called a *bud*) from the side of the chest (figure 2.3). The embryo is a mere 4 millimeters (less than one-sixth of an inch) in length at this time, about the length of a grain of rice. By day 30, the hand appears as a solid paddle. During development, some of this tissue dies as the paddle develops into a hand-like structure with individual digits. The entire formation of the upper limb is completed by day 50. The hand as we recognize it—with 4 fingers and a thumb—becomes visible between 6 and 8 weeks after fertilization. It is during the critical second month after fertilization that congenital limb abnormalities first appear. This is also the same period for development of the heart, which explains why many children have both congenital heart and hand conditions.

Several layers of tissue are involved with limb formation, beginning with the outer layer, called the *apical ectodermal ridge*. Without this structure, no limb forms. If this structure is moved to another part of the embryo's body, a limb will begin to form at the new site. Beneath the apical ectodermal ridge are what are called mesoderm layers of the limb bud. Bone, cartilage, and tendons are formed from one type of this mesoderm, while muscles, nerves, and vessels are formed from another type of this mesoderm.

There are three different signaling mechanisms that direct limb development in the various dimensions, enlarging the limb in the upper and lower directions as well as in the side-to-side direction. We also know that motion of the embryo's upper limb is required for proper formation of joints

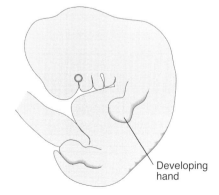

Developing hand

Figure 2.3. The first appearance, during fetal development, of what will become an arm and a hand. ILLUSTRATION BY JACQUELINE SCHAFFER

such as the shoulder, elbow, and wrist. It is no wonder that this complex development sequence can be derailed.

With embryologists' growing knowledge of prenatal development, there was a wave of enthusiasm several years ago for the development of intrauterine surgery to treat conditions and prevent them from causing abnormalities. This idea has not gained widespread acceptance, but converting embryonic research into clinically useful in utero techniques remains a goal in medicine.

GENETICS

One in 626 infants is born with a congenital limb abnormality. One in 10 of these conditions will have a significant impact on the appearance and function of the hand and/or arm. In about half of all cases, the cause of the congenital problem is unknown.

When a genetic basis is identified for the hand difference, it usually falls into one of four categories: the presence of a specific gene or pair of genes that causes the hand defect (a *Mendelian genetic trait*), a chromosomal abnormality, environmental effects on the child's genes, or a combination of influences.

Each of us has 46 chromosomes that occur in 23 pairs. One chromosome in each pair comes from the mother, the other from the father. The first 22 pairs are called *autosomal chromosomes*. Most genes that cause hand abnormalities occur on autosomal chromosomes. The remaining 2 chromosomes are the sex chromosomes. Females have 2 similar sex chromosomes, so-called XX, one from each parent. Males have dissimilar sex chromosomes, an X from the mother and a Y from the father. As of this writing, estimates based on the Human Genome Project place the number of genes on the 46 human chromosomes at 30,000.

DOMINANT VERSUS RECESSIVE GENES

In Mendelian genetics, a trait or characteristic can result from a single dominant gene or a pair of recessive genes. In the case of a single dominant gene, the parent who carries the gene displays the trait, and about half of the children born to this parent will be affected. Examples of congenital hand differences with dominant inheritance are webbed fingers (*syndactyly*) and extra digits (*polydactyly*). In the case of recessive genes, a child will display a trait only if the gene for that trait was received from both parents. The parents often do not display the trait; instead, they carry the recessive gene that they have acquired from one of their own parents and they may or may not pass on the gene to a child. Statistically, hand abnormalities that are the result of recessive genes carried by both parents will affect about one in four of their children. A recessive gene can remain hidden in a family's history, or the condition it causes may skip generations. Hand abnormalities that result from recessive genes are less common but usually more severe than those that result from dominant genes. Many times, hand abnormalities that result from recessive genes involve foot and facial abnormalities as well, such as *Apert syndrome* (a disorder characterized by malformations of the skull, face, hands, and feet.)

Human genetics do not always follow Mendelian principles because multiple genes can be involved in the expression of some traits and because environmental factors may determine whether a particular trait is demonstrated and to what degree. A chromosomal abnormality is the absence, partial absence, or other defect of one chromosome. Chromosomal abnormalities generally appear as syndromes in more than one area of the infant's body. An example is *Down syndrome*, in which affected children have tiny hands with curved, small fingers in addition to intellectual disabilities and cardiac defects.

One thing to remember about genetics is that the risk for each child is the same regardless of how many children in a family have already inherited the genetic disorder. In other words, the risk of inheritance does not decrease with the previous birth of an affected child.

A CLASSIFICATION SYSTEM FOR CONGENITAL HAND DIFFERENCES

In an effort to classify the diverse genetic conditions of the hand, in the early 1970s organizations devoted to hand surgery agreed on an internationally accepted system proposed by Dr. Alfred Swanson, the surgeon who developed the most widely used artificial finger joints. The classification system includes seven groups based on the anatomic appearance of the congenital difference. This system helps treating physicians have more consistent discussions with other surgeons and specialists. The classification system also gives the family a framework for understanding the diversity of congenital differences.

The first category is *failure of upper limb parts to form*. There are two subgroups. The first subgroup is *amputation* at various levels along the upper limb (transverse defects). Amputation in this context does not imply surgical removal; instead, it means absence of a part, such as missing fingers, a missing hand, or a missing hand and part of the arm. This category includes *phocomelia*, which is a deformity in which the hand may be attached to the chest without an intervening upper arm and forearm. Phocomelia was often seen in the late 1950s in the children of mothers who had taken thalidomide, a tranquilizer prescribed for morning sickness, during pregnancy. The other subgroup is *longitudinal defects*, which include defects of the thumb side (radial aspect) of the hand and forearm, defects of the small finger side (ulnar aspect) of the hand and forearm, and defects in the central aspect of the hand, such as the cleft hand.

The second category is *failure of differentiation or separation*, a condition in which the basic hand units are present but not fully or properly developed. The best-known example in this category is webbed fingers (*syndactyly*).

The third category is *duplication*, which refers to the presence of one or more extra digits, including a splitting or duplication of the thumb.

The fourth category is *overgrowth*. This includes enlargement of one or more digits, and is also called *finger gigantism*.

The fifth category, which is paired with the previous category, is *undergrowth* (hypoplasia) of digits, which indicates diminutive size of the digits or the absence of the thumb and fingers.

The sixth category is *constriction band syndrome*, which is caused not by a genetic abnormality of the child but by intrauterine bands (also called *amniotic bands*) that can occur during the development of the fetus and cause constrictions at various levels of the digits and can also involve the rest of the upper limb. Sometimes these constriction bands are so tight that they result in amputation of the fetus's digits or even part of the hand.

The final category is *generalized skeletal abnormalities*. This includes a broad variety of congenital musculoskeletal disorders that do not fit in the previous six categories.

COMMON PROBLEMS

Syndactyly

Syndactyly means webbed fingers, or the congenital joining of two or more fingers in the hand. It is the most common congenital difference, appearing approximately once in every 2,000 births. White infants are affected much more commonly than black infants, at a ratio of 10:1, and male children are affected twice as often as female children.

There are four spaces between the digits of the hand, so-called *web spaces*. The most common web space in syndactyly is the third—between the long and ring fingers. Any web space, however, can be affected. The condition can be inherited as an autosomal dominant trait, appearing regularly in families. It can also be part of a syndrome, in which other health issues appear in the infant. Half the time the condition affects both hands, and half the time the cause cannot be determined.

Particular aspects of the webbing are important to surgeons who treat this condition. The surgeon will want to determine whether the connection between the webbed fingers is incomplete (extending only partway toward the fingertips) or complete (when the two fingers are joined all the way to the tip of the fingers). Before a surgical separation of the fingers can be recommended, it is important to determine whether the fingers are joined only by a skin connection or if there are bone and ligament connections between them. Often, complete syndactylies that go to the tips of the fingers have a shared fingernail.

Surgery is the only remedy for webbed fingers. Although you might think that separation of webbed fingers would be straightforward—with a simple incision between the two fingers—it is not. For one thing, the scar going the length of the finger will contract and shorten when healed (*contracture*), which causes the finger to bend to the side or limits its mobility. Over the years, surgeons have developed techniques to separate the fingers while avoiding scar contracture. Today, there is a standard set of incisions for separating webbed fingers that prevents the surgical scars from impairing the appearance or function of the fingers. Additional skin (a *skin graft*) is usually necessary because once the fingers are separated the existing skin is not sufficient to cover both fingers. Sites for these skin grafts in infants can vary, but most often they are taken from the lower abdomen or outer groin area.

If the syndactyly involves more than two fingers on one hand, only one side of any finger is operated on during a single surgery to protect the artery and maintain blood circulation to the finger. Children who have more than two webbed fingers will need more than one operation for complete separation of all of the involved fingers. The surgery can be done as early as 6 months if the child is healthy and growing, but more commonly the operation is done between 12 and 18 months of age. To prevent inadvertent movement of the hand while this delicate procedure is being carried out, general anesthesia is administered. If there are no other medical issues the surgery is done as an outpatient, same-day operation.

You should expect the surgeon to review with you the risks or complications that can occur. There can be, for example, infection, scars that become thickened or unsightly, a partial recurrence of the webbing between the fingers, or stiffness of the finger joints. Still, the surgery is well-proven and welcomed by parents eager to see their children acquire independent movement of all of fingers.

Extra Digits

Polydactyly is the medical term for extra digits. The most common finger involved is the small finger, and it is the most common congenital abnormality in African Americans, appearing once in every 300 births. When there is an extra small finger, most often the condition is inherited as an autosomal dominant trait and is seen in more than one generation within a family. The extra digit can be just a tiny nubbin or it can be a fully formed finger with mobility, sensation, and fingernail.

The choice of treatment depends on the size and the degree of development of the extra digit. If a small nubbin is present, it is often tied off with a suture or small metallic clip while the newborn is still in the hospital; the nubbin will fall off in about 2 weeks. If the digit is fully formed, the common practice is to wait for the child to reach an age and size when general anesthesia is safe, and then surgically remove the extra digit. During surgery, care is taken to protect the important ligaments and nerves of the hand. After removal of the extra digit, there is usually only a small bump or swelling at the surgical site.

Because thumbs are so important to the function of our hands, extra or "split" thumbs have been extensively studied by hand surgeons. When polydactyly affects the thumb, the two thumbs are not two normal thumbs, side by side. Rather, they are smaller than normal and may have some underlying deficiencies in tendon, nerve, and bone formation. This condition usually affects one hand only, and is not an inherited condition.

There are a number of types of extra thumbs, depending on how many of the three bones that make up the thumb are duplicated. In more than half of the cases, the duplication includes two of the three thumb bones: the bone with the fingernail (*distal phalanx*) and the adjacent bone (*proximal phalanx*). The hand surgeon must evaluate the thumbs to determine which one should remain and which one should be removed. In general, surgeons prefer to keep the thumb that is closest to the other fingers, especially if the width of this thumb is at least 60 percent of the width of the normal thumb on the other hand.

There is no successful nonsurgical treatment for removal of the extra thumb, and surgical treatment is generally carried out before the child is 1 year old. After the surgery, the child will need to be seen by the hand surgeon for several years; as he grows, stiffness, sideways bending, or loose ligaments of the thumb can develop. These conditions can make additional surgery necessary.

Small or Missing Digits

The thumb or any of the fingers can be missing (*aplasia*) or of small size (*hypoplasia*). Intrauterine or amniotic bands that become entangled with the fingers can cause constriction of the circulation and even amputation. Genetic conditions, such as *symbrachydactyly*, which means short, stiff fingers, can also cause this condition. The affected digits can appear as small nubbins or small but normal-looking fingers. There is no nonsurgical treatment because prostheses for individual fingers do not work well.

If the child is born with finger nubbins that have sufficient skin, a surgical procedure called *free toe phalanx grafting* can be performed. This procedure involves taking one bone (a phalanx) from a lesser toe and transferring it into a "pocket" created in the nubbin. If the transfer is done at an early age while the toe's growth center is still active, the toe bone will lengthen in its new location. Joints and knuckles are not transferred in this procedure, but a type of joint can be made to give the child a rudimentary type of finger-bending motion.

If the finger nubbin is not suitable for free toe phalanx grafting, a complete toe transfer can be considered. This complex procedure involves removing an entire lesser toe from the foot, along with the toe's artery, vein, and nerves, and attaching them to the corresponding vessels in the hand to give the new "finger" feeling and function. While the surgery is major, complete toe transfers can allow a child who may have just a single digit in the hand to achieve pinch function (figure 2.4 A, B, C).

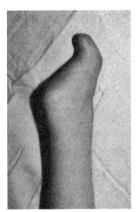 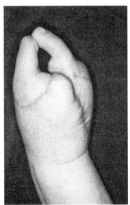 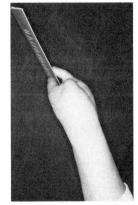

Figure 2.4. Toe transplant. (A) A single digit present at birth of the child; (B) entire toe transferred to the hand with microsurgery; (C) same child using the hand for pinch activity. COURTESY MICHAEL A. MCCLINTON, M.D.

In some children, the thumb may fail to grow properly or be absent. The condition has been divided into four categories, based on the severity of the reduction in size or whether the thumb is present. Type I refers to a thumb that functions normally but is slightly smaller than the normal size. The abnormality of the thumb worsens through types II and III, and at type IV the thumb is barely present or entirely absent. Small thumbs can be part of congenital syndromes that include several abnormalities in the infant, including other musculoskeletal problems, heart defects, and blood clotting disorders. As with small fingers, the small thumb will never "catch up" in size to a normal thumb. The condition can only be addressed with surgery.

Treatment is tailored to the individual child. Some children may not require any surgical treatment if the slightly small thumb has normal function. A careful review of x-rays, looking especially at the quality of the joints or knuckles, can be helpful in determining how the small thumb will ultimately function. In more serious cases of small thumb size (hypoplasia), the treatment is surgical reconstruction of joint, ligaments, and tendons. If there is severe undergrowth or if the thumb is absent, function can sometimes be restored by rotating the adjacent index finger into the thumb position, a procedure called *pollicization of the index finger*. This choice can be a very difficult one for parents; their child, who was born without a thumb, would now lose the adjacent index finger. But the human hand cannot achieve ideal function without opposition, or pinching capability, between a digit in the thumb position and the adjacent fingers. Pollicization of the index finger can allow the hand to pinch and grasp, greatly improving its function and the child's quality of life. And, if the surgery has been performed well, people seeing the child after the procedure generally do not even notice that there is a finger missing. "Before" and "after" photographs of children who have had a pollicization procedure can give parents an idea of what to expect from this procedure.

How the child with the short thumb uses her hand is one factor in predicting the value of pollicization. If, for example, the child does not try to pinch between the abnormal thumb and the rest of the hand but rather uses the index and long finger to pinch, it is unlikely that the thumb will ever be used in regular activities.

Dr. Dieter Buck-Gramcko, a German hand surgeon, was practicing in the late 1950s and early 1960s when thousands of infants were born with thalidomide-induced arm abnormalities. He treated many of the affected infants, including hundreds who were born without a thumb. He performed more than 230 pollicization procedures and made many refinements in the technique. He suggested that the procedure could be performed as early as 6 months. Additional studies by other hand surgeons indicate that children as old as 7 to 10 years are also able to use the new thumb in normal pinch-type activities.

Parents should not, however, expect completely normal function from the new thumb. In general, some stiffness will always be present and strength averages only about 25 percent of a fully functional thumb.

The pollicization procedure is preferred for reconstructing a thumb for the child born with four fingers but no thumb. In the case of fewer than four fingers, the surgeon may recommend microsurgery to transfer one of the lesser toes to the thumb position. Nerves, tendons, and blood vessels are transferred with the toe, and it can provide many of the functions of a thumb, even if it does not look like a normal thumb.

Large Digits (Macrodactyly, or Gigantism)

The normal genetic sequence determines the rate of growth and ultimate size of each individual finger, the relative size of fingers on the same hand, and the symmetry of the digits of both right and left hands. If the genetic sequence is altered, or if the fingers are affected by certain tumors, the fingers or thumb may become enlarged, sometimes to a tremendous degree. *Macrodactyly*, or *gigantism*, is uncommon. When it does occur, it usually involves one extremity and is more common on the thumb/index finger rather than the ring finger/small finger side of the hand. The cause of this condition is not known, but common threads in these cases are overgrowth of the nerve supply to the fingers, overgrowth of finger bones, or tumors.

Treatment of severe digital enlargement is usually only considered when the finger becomes significantly larger than the adjacent fingers. An estimation of the appropriate size for the finger when the child reaches adulthood is determined by comparing it to the size of a parent's finger. (For a female child, comparison would be to the mother's finger; for a male child, it would be to the father's finger.) Affected fingers not only enlarge but also (because they often deviate toward the thumb or small finger) interfere with function of the entire hand. Abnormal lengthening of a finger can sometimes be stopped by surgically disrupting the finger's growth plates. Occasionally, additional procedures to keep adjacent digits from overgrowing and to maintain finger function are necessary as the child grows.

Lack of growth plates does not prevent the finger from enlarging in circumference. Procedures have been described for splitting the finger to keep it small, but these operations often are unsatisfactory. If the surgical treatment is not successful, the enlarged fingers can continue to grow and become very unsightly. Removal of the finger by surgical amputation often is the best functional and cosmetic choice, although it is of course an extremely difficult decision for parents to make.

Radial Deficiency

Radial deficiency (formerly called *radial club hand*) is a term that describes failure of development of the thumb or radial side of the hand and forearm. It is a relatively uncommon condition, appearing only once in 50,000 births. About 25 percent of radial deficiencies are associated with other conditions or syndromes and often these syndromes include heart defects as part of their makeup. *Fanconi anemia*, a rare disorder involving bone marrow failure, may also be connected to radial deficiency. An infant with Fanconi anemia does not make a normal number of blood cells, including the cells that promote proper blood clotting. This condition must be identified before any surgical treatment is undertaken because uncontrolled bleeding or hemorrhage could occur during an operation.

As with small (hypoplastic) thumbs, the classification system for radial deficiency includes four categories. The first category (type I) denotes a slightly smaller radial side of the hand and forearm, and type IV means that the entire radius (the major forearm bone) is absent. Along with underdevelopment of the radial side of the hand and forearm, these children can have smaller, shortened upper-arm bones; bowing of the forearm; abnormalities of the wrist (including extreme thumb-side or radial angulation); stiffness of the fingers; and poorly developed muscles, nerves, and even arteries on the thumb side of the hand. The thumb is rarely normal in these children, and often the status of the thumb determines how much useful function the child will get from the hand.

There is a nonsurgical treatment for radial deficiency. Beginning when the child is very young, splinting or plaster casting can be used to correct or improve bending of the hand on the wrist. In mild cases, this may be the only treatment necessary. In severe cases, this may be a helpful preliminary step before surgical treatment.

Another preliminary step is the use of the *Ilizarov technique*. Gavril Abramovich Ilizarov, a Russian surgeon working in relative obscurity during the communist regime, developed a technique for straightening and lengthening deformed and shortened limbs after a birth deformity or injury. The technique involves a carefully determined cut across the affected bone. Tension is then applied slowly and in a controlled manner to lengthen or straighten the bone. In the case of radial deficiency, the radius forearm bone is divided and an external frame that looks somewhat like an Erector set is applied to the bone. Over a course of several weeks, tension is applied to straighten the angulated bone. This is helpful to prepare for a later surgical procedure that involves centralizing or moving the hand from a significantly angulated position to its proper position at the end of the forearm. This surgical procedure is performed through two incisions, dividing the tight structures that caused the deformity on the thumb side of the hand and wrist, and transferring tendons to the small finger side of the hand to maintain the correction. After surgery, a plaster cast is worn for 3 to 6 months to prevent the forearm from bending. The cast creates stiffness of the wrist but produces far better appearance and, eventually, function for the hand. Called the *centralization procedure*, it is usually done 6 to 18 months after birth.

There is an important caveat that makes straightening the wrist a poor choice in certain children. If the elbow is stiff and does not bend, the only way the child is able to get her hand to her mouth is by the extreme angulation or bending of the wrist. If the wrist is straightened and stiffened and the elbow is also stiff, the child would no longer be able raise her hand to her mouth or face, and function is worsened.

In 75 percent of children who have radial deficiency, the thumb is quite abnormal and requires treatment, usually in the form of pollicization of the index finger. Pollicization is generally carried out after straightening the forearm and wrist.

Phocomelia: The Thalidomide Effect

A person with *phocomelia* has a unique appearance; he has what appears to be a normal hand, but it is connected by a very short or absent forearm and upper arm to the torso. These individuals have virtually no function in their hands and may resort to using their feet to manipulate objects in their environment. Virtually all cases of phocomelia are the result of the mother's use of the drug thalidomide during pregnancy.

Thalidomide, developed in Germany and sold from 1957 to 1961, was intended to reduce morning sickness for pregnant women. Only after the drug resulted in somewhere between 10,000 to 20,000 children born in Europe and Great Britain with major abnormalities of the upper limbs was the connection made and thalidomide taken off the market. In the United States, the effect on children was minimized thanks to the efforts of two women who kept the drug from being released for widespread use. Frances Oldham Kelsey, a pharmacist working at the Food and Drug Administration, and Helen B. Taussig, a pediatric cardiologist at Johns Hopkins Hospital, were both concerned enough about the safety of the drug to campaign against its sale in the United States. As a result, only 17 children suffered the disfiguring effects. Sadly, there is very little reconstruction that can be done for these deformed limbs, although the use of a prosthesis is sometimes possible.

Mat Fraser is a person affected by thalidomide who became a British playwright and actor. In 2005, he wrote and starred in a musical about a person affected by thalidomide. Several other children of the thalidomide epidemic have become lecturers and writers, dedicated to keeping the episode in the public's consciousness and so prevent future tragedies of a similar nature.

Cleft Hand

Cleft hand, as it used to be called, is now known as *central longitudinal deficiency.* As the word *cleft* suggests, these children are born with small or absent digits in the central part of the hand. In the most extreme example, there are single digits on either side of the cleft.

There are two main types of cleft hand. A "true" cleft hand appears to have a "V" in the middle of the hand. It is often bilateral. It is an autosomal dominant trait passed on from parent to child, and it can be associated with cleft lip or cleft palate. The other type of cleft hand has more of a "U"-shaped cleft in the middle of the hand, and it seems to be a different condition; it may include very small nubbins as a residual of the fingers that failed to develop. It is not inherited. Children with cleft hand can function quite well if they have a functioning thumb and are able to pinch and oppose to the small-finger side of the hand.

To make the most of an opposable thumb, one must have an adequate web space or distance between the thumb and the rest of the hand. Some children born with cleft hand have webbing between the thumb and the adjacent index finger that impairs opposition function. A surgical procedure can release the webbing between the digits. Another option, usually performed at 1 to 2 years of age, is to transfer the index finger to the ulnar side of the hand (the side by the little finger), thereby closing the central cleft and opening a web space between the thumb and the fingers.

Sometimes a cleft hand includes only a thumb; all the fingers are missing. In that case, serious consideration is given to a microsurgical transfer of one or two of the toes to provide a movable post to which the thumb can pinch. For this condition or any other categorized as a cleft hand, a great deal of thought must be given before deciding on surgery for the child. Although its appearance can be startling at first, a cleft hand often functions quite well. A hand surgeon never considers surgery to improve cosmetic appearance if the hand's function would be reduced.

◆

In the chapters ahead, you will read about individuals who, despite being born with significant hand abnormalities, went on to live full lives, achieving more than most of us ever will. I hope those stories inspire you. Parents of a child with a hand or arm abnormality may be inspired by the advice of Jim Abbott, the Major League ballplayer (born with no right hand) you read about at the beginning of this chapter. "Treat your kids as normally as possible," Abbott said. "Encourage participation . . . The focus has to remain on what has been given, not what has been taken away."

CHAPTER 3

IT'S ONLY A GAME

◆

The Athlete's Hand

W. Hugh Baugher, M.D., and Thomas J. Graham, M.D.

In 2012, Josh Reddick, a professional baseball player in his first season with the Oakland Athletics (better known as the Oakland A's), was named winner of the American League Gold Glove Award. He had arrived in Oakland after 6 years with the Boston Red Sox, and for a 25-year-old kid who had been in love with baseball his whole life, things couldn't get much better. He finished the 2012 season with 32 home runs and 85 RBIs (runs batted in). Thanks to what manager Bob Melvin called Reddick's "rocket right arm," he led the Oakland A's to the American League Division Series.

The following year, barely a month into the season, Reddick was forced off the field by an injury; he had slammed into the wall while chasing a foul ball. He hit the wall so hard, the impact fractured his right wrist. Placed on the 15-day disabled list, he was left to follow a regimen of rest and physical therapy, hopeful not to miss too much of the 2013 season. If necessary, "surgery is a realistic option," he told a reporter. And he should know; in 2011, after the season ended, he had surgery to repair torn cartilage in his left wrist. Recovery took 2 months, but the procedure and subsequent physical therapy got him back in the game.

Such are the highs and lows of life as a professional athlete. But

Reddick seems able to maintain a calm, optimistic perspective through it all. *How does he do it?* his fans wonder. Reddick credits his parents.

At the beginning of the 2012 season, months before Reddick would be awarded the Gold Glove, the *Mercury News* ran a story about him with this headline: "Oakland A's slugger Josh Reddick gets resilience from father." The reporter, Dan Brown, could not have known that Reddick would achieve one of baseball's pinnacles later that year or the irony that he would do so at the exact same age his father had been when he lost a hand in a horrible accident at work.

In 1988, Kenny Reddick was 25 and working for a power company in Savannah, Georgia. He was married and had two sons; one of them was the not-yet-1-year-old Josh. After a lunch break, Kenny returned to his job site where, without his knowledge, power had been restored to the high-voltage line he'd been working on that morning. The massive jolt of 7,620 volts of electricity nearly killed him (he was pronounced dead 3 times) and inflicted massive burns. His left hand and part of his forearm had to be amputated, and he lost three fingers from his right hand. Many surgeries later, he taught himself to use the end of his left arm and his right hand together to throw a baseball again, to catch, and to swing a bat. (He credits watching a nature video about squirrels for helping him figure out how to do this.) He eventually became a baseball coach—for his sons as well as many other children in the Savannah area.

"Anybody who knows my dad's story can understand the concept of never giving up and not letting stuff get in your way," Reddick says.

Athletes, from the professional to the weekend warrior, are particularly subject to hand injuries by virtue of how engaged the hand is in most sports. To be successful at virtually any sport, be it baseball, football, golf, tennis, archery, or cycling (to name only a few), one must have usable hands. While each sport engages the hand in unique ways and with varying levels of force, hand strength and dexterity play a pivotal role in all of them. Think about a football lineman who uses his hands to outmaneuver his opponent or the adept basketball defender who uses her hands to excel. Even soccer players are hampered when playing with a hand or wrist injury; balance is affected and, if pain is a factor, concentration is, too.

For the professional athlete, a hand injury can be disastrous—

signaling the abrupt end of a hard-fought career, the beginning of income uncertainty (temporary or permanent), and the onset of grief at being forced to abandon a passion. For the rest of us who simply enjoy participating in a sport for fun with friends, a hand injury can be deeply unsettling and will mean, at the very least, an interruption of that activity. At the worst, it can mean much more: medical expenses, lost work time, surgery and recuperation, an inability to carry out responsibilities at home, and so on. For any athlete, professional or otherwise, the questions are the same: *Can it be fixed? Will I have a permanent problem? How will the injury affect my job? How long will it take to get better?*

Just as the hand plays a pivotal role in our day-to-day living, it also serves as a primary tool when we participate in sports. For professional athletes, playing sports is daily life and how a living is made. For them, "perfect" hand and wrist function is central to their profession, their livelihood.

Despite the hand's central role in sports and the impact of its dysfunction, hand or wrist problems in celebrity athletes are largely downplayed as "minor" incidents. A pulled tendon in the finger or a wrist sprain never seems to get the media attention that a tear to the anterior cruciate ligament (ACL) in the knee or a concussion does, but these seemingly small injuries can mean an athlete is unable to fully participate—or play at all. When a team player is out due to an injury, it can mean the difference between winning and losing. When a solo player (golf, tennis) is out with an injury, it can signal the end of a career.

The challenge hand surgeons and any physician caring for an athlete face is the pressure to minimize lost days of play and to return the injured player to the game as rapidly as possible.

TREATING THE PROFESSIONAL ATHLETE

Treatment of the exact same hand injury may be handled differently for an in-season athlete and for an athlete injured during the off-season. The athlete and physician together need to consider the player's short-, medium-, and long-term career and life goals while weighing the risks and benefits of various treatment options.

Injuries and Treatment Choices Viewed
from the Short-Term Perspective

For a professional athlete, "short-term" refers to a single season or what remains in the current one. The immediate concerns when there has been a hand or wrist injury are whether the athlete will be safe (and effective) if he returns to competition that season. A ligament injury in the wrist or hand of a baseball player can often mean the player will return in the same season—after rest, immobilization, or surgery.

When viewing treatment options that might allow a player to return to the game that same season, the big concern is whether deferring surgery or other definitive treatment until after the season has ended will result in a less-than-optimal outcome for the athlete. One way to determine appropriate care in short-term circumstances is to ask how the athlete would be treated if it were the off-season, or if the player was at the end of her career. This kind of analysis can really put things in perspective quickly.

Some professional athletes are emphatic about remaining in the line-up regardless of how an injury is treated. As people who rely on their bodies to make a living, they have usually done their "homework" on surgeons and procedures. They know colleagues who have had similar injuries and they know how soon after surgery they were back in the game. A doctor who proposes a more conservative approach can expect to be challenged. But ultimately, the surgeon must share an honest assessment with the player as to whether he is better off "playing fixed" (returning to the game after surgery and physical therapy). Should a defensive tackle have his scaphoid (wrist) fracture fixed when the injury occurred in the third week of the season, or would it be better to wait until after the end of the play-offs, 4 months later? Some injuries (and a fractured scaphoid is one of them) can safely be left to fix after the season ends, without the athlete missing playing time during the season.

Advances in surgical science and technology have altered the definitions of *aggressive* and *conservative* short-term treatment. Surgery can no longer automatically be considered aggressive or casting considered conservative. For the hand surgeon and the athlete, the primary focus is determining the safest and most effective treatments that will return the player to the game that season. Today, if the surgeon believes that restoring the damaged anatomy and creating a favorable biomechanical environment for healing can be accomplished (and adequately protected through time off or the use of splints and casts), performing surgery in order to return an athlete to the game in-season is a sound decision.

Injuries and Treatment Choices Viewed from the Medium-Term Perspective

While "short-term" is defined as a single season, "medium-term" refers to the expected length of a player's career. (Keep in mind, for professional athletes a "full career" may mean playing until age 40—and for some sports, that would be unrealistically "old.") Like so many other professionals, athletes enjoy not only their beloved sports but also the entire way of life supported by the sports. Leaving the camaraderie of the team as well as the celebrity status and its perquisites is not an easy thing to do. Many players, even after an injury, crave one more championship or league record or particular personal milestone. From the athlete's perspective, these are all legitimate reasons to "hang on for another year." Players also want their children to see them in action, and this desire is no less legitimate than any other.

All of these factors add up to the demand for a special kind of decision-making when an injury occurs at or near the end of a playing career. With the exception of football, however, major North American sports offer guaranteed contracts, which creates a strong incentive for the player to continue participating, even if an injury causes suboptimal performance. When considering the athlete's potential remaining career, the athlete and the surgeon must determine if a particular treatment and its anticipated outcome will no longer even be realistic if he waits to undergo it.

Fortunately, there are few injuries where continued participation would bring about potentially catastrophic consequences, such as chronic *scapholunate dissociation* (an uncorrected wrist injury) or severe *vasospastic disease* (decreased circulation as a response to cold) for winter sports athletes.

Injuries and Treatment Choices Viewed from the Long-Term Perspective

In the life of a professional athlete, "long-term" is defined as life after the career in sports is over. In some sports, like football, where average careers are as short as 2 to 3 years, "life after retirement" will be most of an adult life. With all the big money at stake in professional sports today, and all the pressure on athletes to perform through the pain, someone (besides the player's loved ones) should be looking out for his long-term welfare. Someone needs to be thinking about ensuring that he can enjoy the rest of his life after his sport's career ends.

Hand surgeons do not face discussions like whether the boxer with retinal detachment should fight a final time or whether the linebacker with cervical spine issues or multiple concussions should end his career. Hand surgeons are called on to decide between treatment and "educated neglect" of a particular injury. Which is the best choice, being mindful that the wrong decision may bring about accelerated arthritis or limited motion that could affect the player's hand over the decades ahead?

Sometimes it is more appropriate to treat an injury or disorder after retirement rather than during the player's time of maximal earning potential. Shoulder injuries are good examples of this. Currently, players in the National Football League commonly play with shoulder injuries that will be repaired once they retire. Ed Reed, a linebacker with the Baltimore Ravens who continued playing in 2012 with a torn shoulder labrum, is one such player.

THE ATHLETIC "LABORATORY"

Elite athletes make the perfect "laboratory" for medical treatments and therapies. They are in amazing physical condition, have extraordinary reasons to be compliant with the required protocols, and have every resource needed to assist in their rehabilitation. As a result, surgeons caring for professional athletes can sometimes develop treatments that will eventually be adapted for general use. A couple of examples are early fixation of wrist fractures and pinning of hand fractures; these are two procedures that were originally reserved for athletes but that have translated well into regular application for the general public.

In 1995, the professional baseball player Ken Griffey Jr. fractured his left wrist when he crashed into the centerfield wall during a game. His surgeon used a metal plate and screws to repair the injury, which gave his wrist the stability to allow him to return to play. He continued his successful baseball career until 2010. That technique for fixing wrist fractures is now routinely used on non-athletes as well.

THE AMATEUR ATHLETE

Hand and upper extremity injuries are extremely common in amateur sports events. The hand is used to protect a player, to grab other players, and to manipulate objects—balls, sticks, bats, rackets, and so on. The hand and arm frequently absorb the impact of a collision or a fall. Because the amateur athlete is often able to continue playing with a hand injury, though with reduced effectiveness, these problems are frequently ignored, only to become worse than if they had been treated immediately.

Often, the initial hand injury appears small, but if left untreated what may have been successfully cared for with minimal intervention becomes a problem that may never resolve completely or that may require much more extensive treatment. A ligament injury in the thumb, a common football injury, is a good example. If the player does not wear a splint to avoid further injury, the damage could progress to arthritis. This type of scenario is particularly true in the younger, poorly supervised athlete.

Most hand injuries in athletics are *closed* (this is medical terminology for *internal*, not breaking the skin) and can be treated, at least initially, by nonsurgical methods. But it is important to recognize the injuries that may require more aggressive treatment for optimal outcome. The key to getting proper care for any hand injury is early diagnosis and treatment.

For a person to continue to play with an injury, hand surgeons monitor three parameters. The player's *safety* is the first and most important concern. The hand surgeon must determine whether a player, once appropriately immobilized or splinted, can continue in the game without great risk of doing further damage.

The athlete's *desire* to continue in sports is the second most important concern. This is a judgment that is based on the athlete's status on the team and in life overall. For instance, it would be inappropriate for a Little Leaguer who has a future as a pianist to continue playing baseball after a hand injury; the situation may be quite different for a scholarship athlete who intends to play professional sports. The surgeon's recommendation should be made based on conversations with the coach, the family, and the athlete. Frequently, the coaching staff may decide that the athlete, now only able to complete at a diminished capacity, is not as effective as his backup or substitute, and the decision is made for him.

Parents, coaches, and physicians need to work together to find a solution for the injured athlete, even if it means the player must rest during practice or competition. Feeling invincible is a frequent misconception of the young, which is why it is particularly important for older, wiser heads to prevail when an enthusiastic young athlete is determined to play with an injury. Leaders in healthcare and fitness have launched the STOP (Sports Trauma and Overuse Prevention) sport injuries campaign to educate athletes, parents, trainers, coaches, and healthcare providers about the rapid rise in youth sports injuries and about the necessary steps to keep young athletes healthy. (Learn more at www .STOPSportsinjuries.org.) High school athletes account for an estimated 2 million injuries, 500,000 doctor visits, and 30,000 hospitalizations every year. Overuse injuries are now responsible for nearly half of all sports injuries to middle school and senior high school students. According to the American Academy of Orthopaedic Surgeons, 20 percent of children ages 8 to 12 and 45 percent of those ages 13 to 14 will have arm pain during a single youth baseball season. Little League Baseball has established rest guidelines for pitchers because young pitchers who pitch past the point of fatigue are more likely to end up on the surgery table than those who know when it's time to rest. Prevention of and recovery from hand injuries improve the athlete's chances of continuing to enjoy sports activities throughout life.

The third parameter is the *complexity of the injury* and, if untreated, its effect on other uninjured joints. For instance, a hand injury can change the mechanics of the elbow and shoulder motion. If the athlete protects the injured part, the mechanics of other areas could be altered, producing further problems.

SPECIFIC ATHLETIC INJURIES IN THE HAND

DIP Joint

The DIP joint, or *distal interphalangeal joint*, is the end joint of the finger, or digit (see figure 1.1). It is most commonly injured on the back of the hand, known as the *extensor*, or *dorsal*, surface. The most common injury is called *mallet finger*, otherwise known as a *baseball finger*. The injury occurs when the tendon is torn after the finger is forcibly bent down while the tendon is holding it in a straight or extended position. This results in a tear of the tendon, and the finger hangs in a flexed position. It is often painless and although the injured person cannot straighten the finger on command, it can be passively straightened by applying gentle pressure.

After a DIP joint injury, x-rays should be taken to make sure there is not also a fracture; that information could change the treatment. That said, even relatively large fractures that don't result in partial dislocation of the joint are often treated with just a splint holding the finger straight. It is important for the athlete to understand that the finger must be held in extension for approximately 6 weeks without it bending at all during that time. A pre-fitted splint is often available in the physician's office, but with the help of a good hand therapist, splints can be made that will allow some athletes to continue their sport.

Damage to the palm side of the DIP joint is much less common and can mean a tear of the flexor profundus tendon of the joint, which makes flexion of the finger weak. This kind of injury can happen during football when one player grabs another player's jersey. Swelling often holds the finger slightly flexed at the DIP joint and the tendon itself may retract. At times, the tendon can retract as far as the palm. This injury usually requires surgery to reattach the tendon and it should be fixed early on to obtain the best outcome.

PIP Joint

The PIP, or *proximal interphalangeal, joint*, which is the middle joint of the finger, is a very complex joint and probably the one most commonly injured in the hand (see figure 1.1). A "jammed finger" is usually an injury to the ligament, but with a jammed finger, any significant force or pressure applied to the tip of the finger can result in an injury to the joint, so it is imperative to protect the hand while seeking immediate medical care. The internal ligamentous structures are at risk of tearing, partial tearing, or a complete dislocation of the joint. These joints are usually immobilized temporarily, but it is worthwhile to keep in mind that far more PIP joint injuries are complicated by stiffness than by instability. Thus, protected motion is the most appropriate way to treat many of these injuries. A fracture can also be part of the injury, which is why an x-ray should be taken (figure 3.1). The hand surgeon evaluates the ligaments by stressing them so that appropriate splinting can be used.

There are other injuries that can occur at the PIP joint, such as a complete dislocation of the stabilizing tendons as well as the ligament. These cases may require surgery. For the average PIP joint sprain, standard treatment is a brief period of immobilization of the joint to manage pain and control swelling, but rapidly moving into protected range of motion of the joint. Often, as the joint begins healing, *buddy taping* (taping one finger to another) is an excellent solution for players (figure 3.2), but various hinged splints may be tried as well.

MCP Joint

Injuries to the MCP, or *metacarpophalangeal*, joints (the knuckles) in athletics are relatively common and in many situations, if properly treated, the athlete can continue to participate in her sport. The MCP joints have stabilizing *collateral* (side) ligaments just like the other joints, but are loose when extended and tight when flexed. If a longitudinal load is applied to these joints, such as happens when a person falls on an outstretched hand or is struck by a baseball on the end of a finger, and the joint is sore and swollen, the best way to determine the joint's stability is to flex it—to test its side-to-side stability in a flexed position. Once the

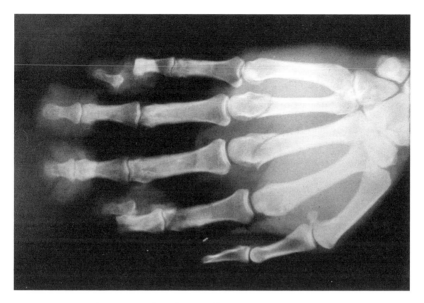

Figure 3.1. X-ray showing combined DIPJ and PIPJ. COURTESY THE CURTIS NATIONAL HAND CENTER

possibility of a fracture is ruled out and it is determined that the injury is to the ligaments or a small bony avulsion (a small piece of bone is torn away with the ligament but does not require replacement surgery), it can be treated with buddy taping or a small hand-based splint to tether the involved joints. If the injury is appropriately padded, many sports, particularly baseball and football, can be resumed and still allow the joint to heal with a splint; sometimes, the fingers can simply be taped for activity (see figure 3.2). True dislocations

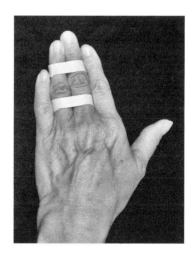

Figure 3.2. Buddy taping. COURTESY NORMAN H. DUBIN, PH.D.

of the MCP joints are rare, but occasionally, when the ligaments become caught in the joint making it impossible to realign, surgery is necessary. If the dislocated joint is not easily placed into proper position, it should be splinted and x-rayed; it may require surgical treatment.

Injuries to the thumb MCP joint are unique because with a tear of the ulnar collateral ligament of the thumb, which is a common occurrence, the ligament can be displaced and will need to be reattached surgically. This sports injury is probably the one that has been understood the longest time. It has been described in the past as "gamekeepers' injury" from the chronic injury seen when a British gamekeeper would stretch this ligament by breaking the neck of a wounded animal over the edge of his thumb. An injury to this joint makes it difficult to pinch with the thumb and, therefore, the injury must be corrected. In sports, this injury occurs most often in football, when a player falls on the thumb, bends the thumb away from the hand, and breaks the ligament that normally holds the thumb in a straight position. This injury also occurs when a hockey player takes off his gloves to fight and bends the thumb away from the hand, or when a skier falls or catches the thumb in the ski pole strap and twists it.

Although there are cases where milder or incomplete tears of the MCP joint injury can be treated without surgery, if there is a complete tear of the ligament with gross instability, an operation will be necessary. If these injuries are neglected, a later surgery can use a ligament graft but the ability to perform daily tasks of living will still be affected, which is why urgent surgery is the best course of action. Dislocations of the thumb joint can sometimes result in an irreducible dislocation if the first attempt at correction is not done carefully. Once the thumb is repaired and swelling has been controlled, the player may resume sports in a custom-molded splint and then progress to tape as the injury becomes more stable.

Injuries to the Wrist

Nerve compression injuries, such as carpal tunnel syndrome (discussed in detail in chapter 9), are relatively uncommon in athletic events, but contusions to the nerves can occur. In long-distance cycling, for example, when the cyclist rests the ulnar aspect of the hand on the handlebars, numbness in the ring and little fingers can occur as a result of the compression to the nerve. When a cyclist experiences this kind of numbness, initial attempts at treatment should be conservative and start with special padding in the gloves, along with rest. If the nerve is severely involved, however, and conservative management does not bring relief, surgical treatment for decompression of the nerve should be considered.

Fractures of the Wrist

Although almost any small bone in the wrist is subject to injury during athletic activities, the more common sports-specific injuries are fractures to the small bones (scaphoid and hook of the hamate). The scaphoid bone bridges two rows of the wrist bones. It has a somewhat tenuous blood supply and is an important bone for wrist stability; it is frequently referred to as "the key" to the wrist. Over time, an untreated fracture of this bone can result in arthritis. On occasion, the initial x-ray may not show the fracture, so when there is an injury to the wrist and pain in the "snuff box" (the spot between your thumb and index finger), the sports physician should have a strong suspicion of a scaphoid fracture. Failure to diagnose and properly treat this injury will result in serious disability to the athlete's wrist. Often, in a poorly supervised athlete, the fracture is diagnosed as a wrist sprain; the athlete recovers to some degree and continues participating in the game only to develop arthritic problems later.

A fracture of the scaphoid bone usually occurs as the result of a fall on the outstretched wrist. If the fracture is non-displaced, a thumb splint is the appropriate treatment. Another option is surgical intervention and internal fixation with a screw. Surgery can sometimes allow an earlier return to sports. There are risks and benefits to both surgical and nonsurgical treatment and both must be carefully evaluated when making this decision. As new cast and splint materials are developed, more and more players are allowed the option of playing in a cast or a splint. Playing in a cast can increase the risk of failure to heal, however—and addressing a failure to heal will require surgery. The athlete must also understand that 3 to 4 months is not an unusual amount of time for a scaphoid fracture to fully heal.

Hamate Fractures

The hook of the hamate bone on the heel of the hand (see figure 1.1) is subject to injury in sports. Many structures in the hand are anchored by the hook of the hamate. The flexor tendons and one of the major nerves and arteries of the hand pass closely by. Their proximity to this bone means the tendons, nerves, or arteries can be irritated when it is injured.

A fracture of the hook of the hamate can result from a direct fall onto the heel of the hand, but it can also occur from injuries sustained when swinging a baseball bat, a golf club, a lacrosse stick, or a tennis racket—whenever the bat or implement acts as a lever, its torque can cause a fracture of this bone. The athlete will complain of pain in the wrist and weakness of grip and occasionally will have symptoms in the flexor tendons or the ulnar nerve. If the player has a history of an injury or the hand is tender to pressure over the hook of the hamate, it's likely the bone has been fractured. Unfortunately, this injury is difficult to see on standard x-rays. CT (computed tomography) scans do show this part of the wrist more clearly but the patient can be in pain during this exam, which limits its usefulness. While more time-consuming and expensive, MRI (magnetic resonance imaging) scans do a good job in showing a hook of the hamate fracture. Sometimes, the fracture can be padded and casted and the athlete can be allowed limited return to play, but most of the time the prognosis for full healing is so poor the hook of the hamate must be removed. While this news startles most people, it can be reassuring to know that many professional baseball players, hockey players, and golfers have had this surgery and are still participating in their sports.

Injuries to the Ligaments of the Wrist

Although ligamentous injuries of any type can occur during athletic events, the most commonly seen sports-specific injury is to the *triangular fibrocartilage complex* (TFCC) on the outer surface of the wrist (see figure 1.1). The TFCC is also often associated with a tendon that lies near this area, responsible for extending the wrist. A twisting injury or impact injury to the wrist can tear or dislocate this ligament. The TFCC cannot be seen on standard x-rays and is best evaluated with the use of a high-field-strength MRI. When there is an injury to the wrist's TFCC ligament, it sometimes can heal with immobilization. A splint or a cast that blocks all wrist motion and rotation must be worn. In some cases surgery is necessary.

Forearm and Elbow Injuries

Strains of the muscles and tendons of the forearm, commonly seen in baseball pitchers, are usually treated by splinting and periods of rest. Another more common problem in the elbow is a tear of the ligaments on the inner aspect of the elbow, which is treated by the so-called Tommy John surgery—reconstructing the ligament with a tendon taken from the forearm. Few athletes and physicians realize that Tommy John, a pitcher for the Yankees, whose Major Baseball League career spanned 26 years (1963 to 1989), had to have two operations to correct the injury. During the initial surgery, a nerve was pinched by scar tissue that built up from the reconstruction, causing severe pain. A second operation was performed to move the nerves into a more appropriate position. Today, the operation includes moving or protecting the nerve when the ligament is reconstructed.

◆

Whether amateur or professional, any athlete who experiences an injury to the hand needs proper, timely care. The goal of the hand specialist is the same in every case: to minimize the effect of the injury so that the person's overall quality of life is not diminished.

CHAPTER 4

WORN DOWN BUT NOT OUT

◆

The Arthritic Hand

Philip Clapham, B.S., and Kevin C. Chung, M.D.

It was a few minutes after midnight on June 22, 1937, at the Chicago White Sox's Comiskey Park when 32-year-old James J. Braddock fell down unconscious in the boxing ring. Braddock, popularly referred to as the "Cinderella Man" because of his rise from the Depression-era slums of New York to the height of boxing fame, was defeated in the eighth round by the up-and-coming 23-year-old Joe Louis. It would be the last highly publicized fight of Braddock's career. Two years earlier, with the betting odds 10 to 1 against him, Braddock had knocked out the defender Max Baer in a 15-round fight at Manhattan's Madison Square Garden and was crowned boxing's new World Heavyweight Champion. That fight, which brought Braddock world renown, is still hailed as the biggest upset in boxing history.

In addition to boxing, Braddock had worked as a longshoreman for years, enduring long days of manual labor at the Manhattan docks. The hazards of those two arduous occupations finally caught up to him and, in the years between the Baer and Louis fights, Braddock experienced a rapid onset of osteoarthritis in his hands.

Osteoarthritis, the most common form of arthritis, is the progressive loss of cartilage within a joint. It is associated with "wear and tear" activities and with age. The symptoms include pain, a loss of mobility, stiffness, and swelling. The person experiencing it often refers to a feeling of "bone on bone" when using the joint, which is a fairly accurate assessment of what x-rays usually reveal.

For Braddock, the pain and stiffness became especially bad in his right hand (his dominant hand). To compensate, he retrained to make his left arm the stronger one. Unfortunately, the arthritis symptoms continued to spread across his upper body and by the night he fought Joe Louis, the mighty Braddock could barely lift his arms above his head. A few months after the fight, Braddock officially retired.

Although arthritis had ended his career as a boxer, James Braddock was by no means incapacitated by it, going on to enlist in the United States Army. After serving and fighting in World War II as a first lieutenant, Braddock worked as a marine equipment supplier in New Jersey, where he lived with his wife until he died in 1974, at age 69.

Like Braddock, many of the 46 million Americans living with some form of arthritis are able to combat the crippling symptoms of their disease. The U.S. Centers for Disease Control and Prevention estimates that arthritis "limits the activities" of 19 million—fewer than half of those affected. The good news today is that many individuals who develop arthritis will remain highly functional and continue to lead productive lives.

For some, however, arthritis is a severely deforming and disabling condition. Because it can affect joints and bones in different areas of the body and cause nearly constant pain, the simple daily activities of life can become challenging. Activities that require the use of the hands can become excruciatingly painful and arduous, and sometimes even impossible. For these individuals, simple tasks—picking up a pen or opening a jar or, as in James Braddock's case, making a fist—are difficult if not impossible.

The general term *arthritis* refers to a broad group of conditions that affects the body's joints and causes pain and difficulty in movement, but there are distinct types of arthritis with different causes and varying symptoms. In this chapter, you will find a description of the causes, physical appearances, and symptoms of the two most common types of arthritis as they relate to the hand—osteoarthritis and rheumatoid arthritis—and what can be done to address them.

As mentioned earlier, *osteoarthritis* is a loss of the cushioning cartilage within a joint; rheumatoid arthritis, although it can have similar symptoms (most notably pain and stiffness), is a completely different disease. *Rheumatoid arthritis* is an autoimmune disorder, in which the immune system is attacking healthy tissue (the opposite of its function), causing chronic inflammation, particularly around the joints, and resulting in a loss of bone.

OSTEOARTHRITIS

Osteoarthritis is the most common arthritic condition, affecting nearly 30 million adults in the United States. It affects the cartilage in the joints, known as *articular cartilage*. Cartilage is a flexible and fibrous tissue in the body's joints that cushions the bones during motion. In individuals with osteoarthritis, this cartilage has worn very thin, allowing the bones in the joint to rub against each other, causing pain and difficulty in movement. The severity of the loss of cartilage varies, which is why many people (like Braddock) are able to adapt to their pain and impairment and adjust their lifestyle to accommodate the symptoms of their disease.

Because we use our hands to do so many things, the joints of the hand experience a lot of stress and are especially vulnerable to injury. In addition, the day-to-day use of our hands causes general "wear and tear" as we age. For this reason, the hands are commonly affected by osteoarthritis. Specifically, the *distal interphalangeal joints* (abbreviated as the DIP joints) of the fingers and the *carpometacarpal joint* (abbreviated as the CMC joint) in the thumb are where osteoarthritic symptoms are most prominently felt (see figure 1.1). Osteoarthritis is fairly common in the wrist joint as well, especially if the wrist has been injured at some point during a person's life.

Development of Osteoarthritis

Within a joint, if the *ligaments* (the tissues that connect and support the bones) are torn as a result of an injury, the normal motion of the joint is altered. When the bones begin to move outside their normal path, they start rubbing against new tissues and other bones that were not made to stand up to these constant stresses. Over time, the repeated abnormal motion of the joint wears down the articular cartilage and the bone is exposed in the joint. The result can be the onset of osteoarthritis. This path to arthritis is most frequently seen in the wrist, where fractures or tears in the ligament that connect the scaphoid and lunate bones of the wrist are common outcomes of traumatic injuries. A tear or fracture here can cause the scaphoid bone to scrape against the radius bone during movement, which is extremely painful. Once the degenerative process begins in one area of the joint, the cartilage is weakened and the "wear and tear" across the remaining surfaces of the joint progresses quickly, causing pain to spread across the entire wrist.

The loss of articular cartilage that is characteristic of osteoarthritis causes pain because the cushion and lubricated surface provided by the cartilage is gone. Imagine the pistons of a car engine moving over and over again through their cylinders without sufficient lubrication. Eventually, chronic chafing of the metal cylinders would lead to a "seized" engine. Similarly, the end result of osteoarthritis is bone rubbing against bone, causing pain that most sufferers describe as a sharp ache or burning sensation. Pain is the primary reason that individuals with osteoarthritis are forced to limit their activities and reduce any movements that require the motion of the affected joints. In this regard, especially for individuals accustomed to more active lifestyles, osteoarthritis can be significantly disabling, even depressing.

Because osteoarthritis is more common in elderly people and in people who engage in manual labor or strenuous activities such as high-impact sports that place a lot of force on particular joints in the body, many people erroneously believe that age and activity-related injury are the only causes of osteoarthritis. In reality, many studies point to a hereditary basis for osteoarthritis, with one study finding that up to 65 percent of those with osteoarthritis have genetic factors that predispose them to the disease. Though age is not a direct cause of osteoarthritis, the water content of cartilage steadily decreases as we age, causing the cartilage to weaken, which is why elderly people experience higher rates of osteoarthritis.

Nonsurgical Treatments for Osteoarthritis of the Hand

Most individuals experiencing osteoarthritis of the hand typically report one or more of the following symptoms:

- joint pain that is especially acute during movement
- swelling of the affected joints
- a "popping out" or "clicking" noise and/or sensation upon joint motion

Because osteoarthritis does not have a single clear cause, medical interventions primarily aim to alleviate the symptoms. You may have read articles in consumer magazines that endorse products such as glucosamine and shark cartilage derivatives as ways to "regenerate cartilage," but none of these treatments have been proven to promote the healing of damaged cartilage or the regeneration of lost tissue. Currently, frontline treatments aim to reduce pain by limiting movement of the affected joint through splinting, or by making movement easier with the use of anti-inflammatory medications like ibuprofen.

Surgical Treatments for Osteoarthritis of the Hand

Although conservative interventions can help address the symptoms of osteoarthritis, symptoms can eventually worsen to a disabling or unbearable state. When that happens, a consultation with a hand surgeon is warranted. There are currently two types of surgical treatment for osteoarthritis: fusion of the joint and joint replacement. The surgery that is best for a particular case is determined by which joint is affected and the extent of the arthritis in that joint. For osteoarthritis of the DIP joint, some hand surgeons recommend fusion. Pinching stresses the DIP joint quite a bit and fusion provides stability, whereas implant replacements of this joint have a tendency to dislocate with sufficient pressure.

In a *fusion* procedure, the surgeon removes the destroyed carti-lage and the joint is pinned in a fixed position for 6 to 8 weeks during which time the bones fuse together. Once fused, a joint will no longer move. This time-honored operation has been proven to result in good outcomes; the finger will be pain-free and the hand's motion is largely maintained because the other joints in that finger still work. In addition, the finger will have a much better aesthetic appearance.

In contrast, for osteoarthritis of the CMC joint (carpometacarpal) joint in the thumb, the most common surgical treatment is the removal of the trapezium followed by a ligament arthroplasty procedure. The trapezium, one of the eight bones in the wrist, has a saddle shape and it sits below the metacarpal bone of the thumb. In this procedure, the arthritic trapezium is removed and a tendon is used to stabilize the CMC joint and mimic the function of a ligament. An *arthroplasty*, which simply means a surgical reconstruction of a joint, will allow the person to maintain good thumb function, highly important because the thumb plays a critical role in so many tasks. Because it would limit the motion of the thumb, fusion is not typically recommended in the CMC joint.

One downside of ligament arthroplasty for the thumb's CMC joint is that this procedure generally requires a long recovery period, even up to a year. For those who engage in manual activities or require good hand strength, the shorter recovery period of a fusion operation, which also gives great stability, may be a more attractive option. The tradeoffs between these two procedures is a subject for discussion with your physician.

A third surgical option for treating osteoarthritis of the hand comes in the form of a fairly new pyrocarbon implant. *Pyrocarbon implant ar-throplasty* is a promising new development but because of concerns for complications such as implant dislocation, outcomes data are still pend-ing to demonstrate its long-term reliability and durability. The two-piece design has been in development for the past 20 years and has been made available in recent years for replacement of joints in the hand. This innovative implant offers a good assimilation of the original, healthy joint, and is designed to have the same shape as the articular surface of the bones. During the operation, the surgeon cuts out the articular surfaces of the bones in the damaged joint and replaces them with the implant. Due to their design, pyrocarbon implants mimic the structure of the joint and give it acceptable functional outcomes while also maintaining stability.

When osteoarthritis affects a person's MCP (*metacarpophalangeal*) or PIP (*proximal interphalangeal*) joints , the tradeoffs between stability and motion need to be carefully considered when choosing surgical treatment. In the thumb's MCP joint, for example, the pinch function requires a great deal of joint stability, so some surgeons recommend fusion rather than arthroplasty. In contrast, MCP joint fusion in the fingers is limiting because that joint's movement is critical for grasping or fist-clenching. Fusion of the MCP joint in the fingers would essentially rob the hand of most of its function because the fingers would be permanently stuck in a particular position. For this reason, implant arthroplasty is the usual treatment for the MCP joint. Although one-piece silicone implants have been used to replace osteoarthritic MCP joints, many hand surgeons now prefer the two-piece pyrocarbon implants because of the better motion they provide. The strong ligaments of the fingers' MCP joints can support the pyrocarbon implants and the two-piece design provides better motion.

For the PIP joint, the choice between arthroplasty and fusion is more complicated. Arthritic PIP joints are common locations for *bone spurs*, little bumps of bony material that form on the bones. Bone spurs can occur as a bone heals after injury, or as a result of rubbing, pressure, or stress. They accumulate as we age. Studies show that pyrocarbon implant arthroplasty of the PIP joint can provide good relief of pain, which is why it is recommended if the primary goal of surgery is to alleviate pain. If the person's desire is increased motion at the PIP joint, however, she will be disappointed because the amount of joint motion after pyrocarbon implant arthroplasty procedure is unpredictable. In addition, the potential of implant dislocation must be considered.

Osteoarthritis is a condition many of us will face as we age. When you are considering treatment for osteoarthritis, it is important to look at all the options. Conservative measures are good first steps but if you eventually find you still have significant pain and difficulty moving your hand, consulting with a hand surgeon about surgical options is the next step. Keep in mind the tradeoffs between stability and movement that are offered by fusion and arthroplasty procedures. It is also important that you have realistic expectations about the likely surgical outcome. Surgical procedures tend to be successful in reducing pain, but regaining full hand function and motion is not possible.

RHEUMATOID ARTHRITIS

Rheumatoid arthritis is an entirely different disease than osteoarthritis. It is a systemic disease, which means it can affect organs and tissues in any part of the body. Rheumatoid arthritis is thought to be caused by an altered immune system, in which the cells of the person's own immune system attack the cells of the synovial lining of the body's joints. The *synovial lining* is a double-ply layer of specialized tissue that surrounds and lines the body's joints. It also produces a lubrication fluid, called *synovial fluid*, which facilitates easy motion of the joint. The synovial tissue creates a closed space around the joint to keep the synovial fluid within the joint. In rheumatoid arthritis, the synovial lining is damaged by the cells of the immune system, causing inflammation and the progressive destruction of the articular cartilage as well as the bone itself. The result is progressively worsening pain and stiffness in the joints, causing motion to be limited.

Development of Rheumatoid Arthritis

Rheumatoid arthritis affects approximately 1.3 million Americans and 3 times as many women as men. Although symptoms sometimes show up in other organs, rheumatoid arthritis primarily affects joints, most commonly those in the hands and feet. Typically, in the initial phases of the disease, a person experiences inflammation and stiffness in the joints, especially upon waking in the morning or following a period of inactivity. Rheumatoid arthritis can be so painful and disabling that within a few years of diagnosis, many sufferers are unable to work.

In the hand, rheumatoid arthritis often causes severe finger or wrist deformities or dislocations. The inflammation of the joint, which stretches and destroys the ligaments and articular cartilage, is the cause of the disfigurement. As a result, rheumatoid arthritis causes difficulty with everyday tasks such as holding utensils, removing the top of a jar, or holding a hair brush.

Just as with osteoarthritis, there are examples of individuals adapting amazingly well to life with rheumatoid arthritis. The nineteenth-century French impressionist painter Pierre Renoir is perhaps the best known. He was a longtime sufferer of rheumatoid arthritis, and for the last 30 years of his life (and painting career) his hands were so contracted he could not pick up a paint brush. He could, however, grip it once it had been placed in his hand, and he produced some of his most famous works during this period of his life.

Nonsurgical Treatments for Rheumatoid Arthritis

Unfortunately, no known cure exists for rheumatoid arthritis and once the damage to the joint has occurred, rheumatoid arthritis is irreversible. There are, however, a variety of treatments that help lessen its symptoms and even slow its progression. Anti-inflammatories and *analgesics* (drugs used to relieve pain) can help with some of the pain and stiffness. To slow the disease's progression, many rheumatologists will prescribe one or more medications known as *disease-modifying antirheumatic drugs* (DMARDs), which act to modify the immune system.

Surgical Treatments for Rheumatoid Arthritis

For many with rheumatoid arthritis, drug therapy is enormously successful in providing relief from the pain and stiffness, and these individuals are able to adapt their day-to-day activities to their new functional abilities. Some, however, suffer from crippling deformities of the fingers and wrists. For these individuals, surgical treatment may be beneficial. A consultation with a rheumatologist can help you decide if an appointment with a hand surgeon is warranted. If surgery is decided upon, the hand surgeon and rheumatologist will work with you to adjust the medications and rehabilitation treatments to achieve the best possible outcome after surgery.

The majority of rheumatoid arthritis cases a hand surgeon sees include a deformity of the ulna at the wrist joint. In this deformity, the ulna protrudes over the back of the hand (referred to as *dorsal subluxation of the ulna*) because the inflammation in the wrist joint loosens the ligaments that support the joint. The rubbing of the end of the ulna against the bones of the wrist can cause extreme pain as well as erosion in the articular surface of the ulna. In severe cases, this deformity can cause the rupture of certain extensor tendons of the wrist as the displaced ulna pushes on them, causing a loss of ability to extend the fingers.

If the extensor tendons are ruptured as a result of dorsal subluxation of the ulna, a hand surgeon has several options to move other tendons in the arm to restore the fingers' abilities. The normal recovery time from these procedures can be quite lengthy, which is why it is always better to operate and correct the deformity before rupture occurs. The most common treatment is the removal of the displaced piece of the ulna to prevent it from rubbing against the other bones in the wrist joint and eliminating the risk of ruptured extensor tendons.

Another common deformity that prompts many with rheumatoid arthritis to seek surgery is the dislocation of the thumb and fingers at the MCP joint (figure 4.1). Once again, this particular deformity is the result of a loosening of the supporting ligaments because of inflammation, a condition that allows the fingers to deviate from their normal settings. Especially in the fingers' MCP joints, rheumatoid arthritis leaves them unstable and the ability to grip and pick up items is greatly compromised. Implant arthroplasty of these joints is a common procedure as it strengthens the weakened joints and corrects the deviation of the fingers. Both the aesthetic appearance of the hand and its function are greatly improved, and studies show good 1-year outcomes.

Like any surgery, the decision is determined by how well the hand functions and by the person's needs. It is critical that the patient work collaboratively with the rheumatologist and the hand surgeon to determine if the deformity has developed to a great enough degree that surgery is warranted. Although restoring full hand function is not a likely outcome, with careful planning, notable improvement can be achieved.

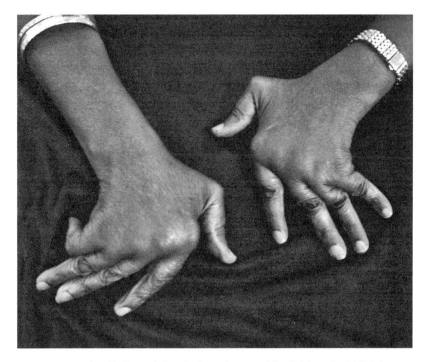

Figure 4.1. Hands with finger deformity from rheumatoid arthritis at the MCP joint.
COURTESY THE CURTIS NATIONAL HAND CENTER

OTHER TYPES OF ARTHRITIS OF THE HAND

There are several rare forms of arthritis that can affect the hand, accounting for less than 1 percent of arthritic conditions. Retained foreign bodies—sea urchin quills, embedded fiberglass strands, and silicone are a few we've seen—produce toxins that can cause inflammatory arthritis in the finger joints.

"Gouty" arthritis, a form of arthritis that is caused by deposits of needle-like crystals of uric acid in the joint spaces, can strike all joints in the hand. The acute inflammation it causes can be confused with infection.

Psoriatic arthritis is a chronic disease characterized by inflammation of the skin (psoriasis) and the joints (arthritis). Approximately 10 percent of people with psoriasis also develop an associated inflammation of their joints, which is diagnosed as psoriatic arthritis. This particular arthritis usually occurs in people in their forties and fifties, and in most cases psoriasis of the skin shows up before the joint disease.

◆

Arthritis of the hands is neither a benign disease nor a condition that we must resign ourselves to as we age. There are a variety of reconstructive surgical procedures that can greatly improve the hand's function and appearance while reducing or eliminating pain. The first step is a consultation with your doctor to determine if there is a surgical option that would be a good choice for you.

CHAPTER 5

GOOD VIBRATIONS

◆

The Musician's Hand

Raymond A. Wittstadt, M.D.

Sarah is a 17-year-old musical prodigy. She began playing the violin at age 4 and is now taking lessons at a prestigious conservatory. In preparation for an upcoming concert, she has been practicing 5 hours a day. For weeks, her forearms have been aching after practice. But now she is finding that the pain flares up during other activities as well, such as writing or using a keyboard. Her family doctor recommended an anti-inflammatory medication but the pain persisted. Next stop: a visit to an orthopedist. That doctor diagnosed tendonitis, prescribed physical therapy (PT), and recommended an extended break from the violin.

After 4 PT sessions over the course of 2 weeks, Sarah was pleased to find the exercises were providing some relief from what had become debilitating pain. But as soon as she picked up the violin, the pain returned. She had to cancel her participation in the concert she had practiced so hard for and is now seriously worried (as are her parents) about upcoming auditions for college applications—she can't play for more than 15 minutes without stopping because of excruciating pain. Massage, acupuncture, herbal treatments—nothing has helped. She is getting desperate. Eventually, her music teacher recommended that she seek out a performing arts medical specialist.

Sarah has a *repetitive motion disorder*, a class of conditions that occur when any biologic tissue, muscle, bone, tendon, or ligament is stressed beyond its physical limits. When the body is not allowed sufficient time to recover from a repeated physical demand, pain sends a message loud and clear: *STOP!* As Dr. Bernardino Ramazzini, an eighteenth-century expert in occupational diseases and a man ahead of his time, noted, "No sort of exercise is so healthful or harmless that it does not cause serious disorders, that is, when overdone."

The occupation of being a professional performing musician requires rapid and controlled repetitive movements and is arguably among the hardest activities one can do with the hands and upper extremities. The intense concentration, motivation, discipline, and prolonged solitary practice required for a musician to reach a professional level are incredibly difficult. Although the extraordinary demands musicians place on their upper limbs seem obvious, when quantified they are astounding. A study in 1977 of a pianist playing a presto (fast) piece composed by Felix Mendelssohn revealed that in 4 minutes and 3 seconds the musician played 5,595 notes and his hands (combined) made 72 finger movements per second.

Until recently, little was written about the injuries performing musicians experience, and only within the past 20 years or so have the health problems of musicians (mostly classical musicians) been the basis of medical studies. A complicating factor in describing and quantifying medical problems specific to musicians is that there is rarely a simple cause and effect. Many unique factors—related to the individual musician and the instrument he plays—can contribute to the development of a variety of painful symptoms.

The largest survey of medical problems specific to musicians was commissioned in 1989 by the International Conference of Symphony and Opera Musicians (ICSOM) of more than 4,000 working musicians. Although keyboard players were underrepresented, this survey is the standard to which all others are still compared. The data revealed a high incidence of significant symptoms. Thirty-six percent (more than 1,400 of the group studied) listed up to 4 severe problems. Eighty-four percent of string players had at least one problem with pain in their upper extremity and of that group 76 percent had symptoms severe enough to compromise their playing. Severe problems were more common in musicians under age 35, but those between 35 and 45 years of age were most likely to report at least one problem. Physical pain was more prevalent among string players, but players of woodwind, brass, and other instruments also reported a high incidence of medical problems.

These are significant data to digest, but what they clearly reveal is that professional performing musicians are subject to a high degree of hand and upper extremity stress and subsequent disorders, many of which become so severe the person is unable to continue her work. Although many of these medical problems have been referred to as repetitive strain disorders, they are neither inevitable nor progressive. Most musicians can avoid problems by following "good" technique, a sensible lifestyle, and some basic physical strength and flexibility conditioning (away from the instrument!).

Musicians with painful symptoms are often reluctant to seek medical care, and many do so only after a considerable period of disability and self-treatment. Fear of job loss, a tradition of "suffering," peer pressure, lack of medical awareness, and limited insurance coverage contribute to delays in seeking treatment. High-level musicianship is, in many ways, similar to high-level athletics. There is lots of competition for these relatively few elevated positions in the music world; reporting injuries, or pain that might limit performance ability, can (and does) result in job loss.

In addition, the response from medical providers—ranging from unhelpful treatments to disbelief—can be very off-putting to musicians seeking medical advice. Complying with the simple advice to "avoid the painful activity" may be impossible. Therapy isolated to the painful area only, without consideration of the entire individual, is often less than successful. Janet Horvath, a world-class cello player, details her problems in her book *Playing Less Hurt*. She sought medical care and suffered a fear of "failure" when she developed pain in her left hand and arm while she was a student at Indiana University. She consulted with a dozen physicians, only to be frustrated by their shrugging and unhelpful responses. Immobilized by pain, fear, and despair, she did not touch her instrument for 3 months. She was reluctant to tell her mentor, the cellist Janos Starker, fearing that her career was over. Fortunately, Starker proved remarkably understanding and proceeded to help Horvath rebuild her technique using a "whole body" approach. Her recovery took 9 months and inspired her to share her experiences in her book.

AT-RISK MUSICIANS

Categorizing the particular medical problems of musicians is still evolving in the medical world but at the moment it is believed that musicians' problems can be designated as one or more of the following three groups:

- damage from rheumatoid arthritis or from other disorders or injuries of the joints, tendons, ligaments, and nerves
- problems directly related to playing the instrument, or of a "technical" nature
- problems induced by psychological and emotional stress, or so-called stage fright

Musculoskeletal problems are grouped into three diagnostic categories. In order of decreasing frequency they are:

- musculoskeletal pain and overuse syndromes
- peripheral neuropathies and nerve entrapment
- *focal dystonias* (neurological conditions that cause involuntary muscular contractions)

Several factors seem to make music students more vulnerable than professional career musicians to performance-related medical problems. Student music camps and summer festivals can lead to injuries due to the sudden increase in playing time during these intense events. For example, a student who usually practices 2 to 3 hours a day may find herself playing 6 to 8 hours a day during a summer camp. The desire to get the most out of these brief events with peers and notable teachers, combined with trying new techniques, can set the stage for injuries. The end of the school year can also bring increased practice time; the stress of competitions, juries, and auditions further heightens the risk of injury for the student musician.

Those students who participate in a marching band expand the possible sites of injuries. The need to hold the musical instrument while marching in a precise manner and playing in cold, damp, or hot weather increases the risk of low back and lower extremity injuries. Although these musicians are an understudied group, it is reasonable to state that the intermittent nature of their playing times also predisposes them to injuries.

The ICSOM study and other current research have provided a clearer picture of the "what, where, and why" of injuries in professional classical musicians: the frequent change of repertoire, varying performance times, and travel across time zones can all contribute to injuries. In addition, the study revealed a relative risk of injury correlated to the type of instrument.

PREDISPOSING FACTORS FOR INJURIES

Overuse injuries occur when a biologic tissue is stressed beyond its physical limit. Such injuries are classified as acute or chronic. Acute symptoms develop after a specific activity, and the musician can usually recall the exact onset of pain. Often, acute symptoms occur after a prolonged practice session or when attempting to master a new technique or passage. Chronic overuse injuries have a more insidious onset, starting with minimal discomfort that worsens over time. Overuse, inconsistent use, and misuse are all potential sources of injury. *The Musician's Survival Manual* lists a dozen factors that can predispose a musician to injury. These apply to the amateur as well as to the professional musician:

- inadequate physical conditioning
- sudden increase in playing time
- errors in practice habits
- errors in technique
- change in instrument
- inadequate rehabilitation of a previous injury
- improper body mechanics and posture

- physically stressful nonmusical activities
- anatomic variations
- gender
- quality of instrument
- environmental factors

Inadequate Physical Conditioning

As a hand surgeon, I frequently see cases where inadequate physical conditioning is the major cause of a musician's injuries. Although musicians tend to be "nonathletic," they need to observe many of the same conditioning steps that athletes follow for injury-free performances. In a way, playing a musical instrument for 3 hours is equivalent to running a marathon with your hands and arms. While proper warm-up and general conditioning are stressed in all athletic activities, they are usually overlooked in musical practice and performance. The problem is that muscles that are weak, poorly conditioned, or excessively tight are prone to overuse injuries.

Sudden Increase in Playing Time

Professional and dedicated student musicians are functioning at the physiologic limits of what their hands can do. Any rapid or sudden change in the amount of practice or playing time is perhaps the most common cause of overuse injuries, as shown by the number of injuries after summer camps. The best way to minimize overuse is to increase playing time gradually, perhaps adding only 10 to 15 minutes to a practice session over a period of days or weeks.

Errors in Practice Habits

As a musician, you need to think of playing an instrument as a total body activity. Many musicians skip warm-ups completely, or consider playing scales or slow passages as enough of a warm-up. Whether it is immediately apparent or not, a musical instrument is played with the entire body, and the entire body must be warmed up in some manner before beginning to play. You will benefit greatly by beginning a practice session with 5 to 10 minutes of an activity that increases your heart rate a little, such as walking up steps, doing jumping jacks, or even doing squat thrusts. The aerobic cardio warm-up should be followed by a few minutes of gentle stretching, particularly of any tight muscles. (Note: if you have joint laxity—so-called double-jointedness or loose joints—be careful not to overstretch your joints and muscles.) Only after a sufficient warm-up should the musician begin to play.

You should avoid continuous practicing of difficult passages. Trying to master a difficult segment or new technique in one long session can lead to overuse injuries. Limiting practice of difficult passages to 5 or 10 minutes at a time, with frequent breaks to play other, less difficult material, can help prevent injuries. Remember: fatigue decreases coordination. Studies reveal that repetitive hand and wrist activities reduce forearm blood flow after 90 minutes; practice continued beyond an hour and a half is counterproductive. All it takes is a quick break of 5 to 10 minutes for rest and gentle stretching to restore normal blood flow. An ideal practice session schedule should look like this: a 10-minute warm-up, 40 minutes of playing, a 10-minute rest or cool down period. This cycle can then be repeated.

Errors in Technique

Excessive tension while playing is a common cause of overuse injuries for a musician. Gripping the instrument or bow too tightly while playing stringed instruments creates extra tension in the muscles and requires additional force and energy that can lead to injuries. Drumsticks, wind instruments, and bows (as well as steering wheels, pens, and cell phones) are commonly gripped harder than necessary. This tension can spread to the musician's shoulder, neck, and back, compounding the potential for overuse injuries. The modern imaging technology used for motion analysis of professional athletes is gradually being accepted in other occupations; for musicians, it would lead to a better understanding of proper muscle tension and technique.

Change in Instrument

Any change to the musician's instrument can contribute to potential injury. Changing the bow or bridge, for instance, or getting new strings (which may require slightly more force to depress), or getting a new instrument can increase stress on the hands and arms. Any change in the instrument, repertoire, or teacher should be accompanied by a modest reduction in playing time to allow your body to adjust.

Inadequate Rehabilitation of a Previous Injury

A return to vigorous playing before complete recovery from an injury can lead to a setback at best, or additional injuries at worst. As a musician, you must continue treatment until you are free of pain, have a full range of motion, and have regained your strength and endurance. This is a challenge for professional musicians, but failure to do so can lead to subtle changes in technique, which in turn can result in new problems.

Improper Body Mechanics and Posture

Poor body posture and mechanics along with inadequate conditioning often underlie many musicians' injuries. Most professional musicians began their training at a young age, while they were still growing; as the body makes accommodations to the instrument, physical changes can result in poor posture and body mechanics. It is also important to pay attention to how the instrument is transported because improper form during that frequent activity can contribute to overuse injuries. Musicians who participate in yoga, Alexander Technique, or Feldenkrais body therapy find it easier to maintain good posture.

Physically Stressful Nonmusical Activities

Nonmusical tasks can contribute to the development of overuse injuries, too. The routine duties of daily life—housecleaning, yard work, school work, or other obligations—can add to the stress on the musician's hand. Hands have only so many contractions in them each day, and the contractions must be distributed evenly among all of the day's activities. On days when other work needs to be done, playing time should be decreased accordingly.

Anatomic Variations

The simple fact is this: not every person can play every instrument. Since many musicians begin training as children, it is impossible to know how well they will ultimately "fit" their chosen instrument.

Many musicians have excessive joint *laxity* (looseness). Other anatomic variations can be abnormal tendon connections or the absence of the superficialis flexor tendon to the small finger. It is not clear if these variations are protective and facilitative for musicians, or a liability for which corrective measures need to be taken. In the general population, for example, only 5 to 6 percent have *benign hypermobility syndrome* (joints move beyond the normal expected range of motion). Among musicians seeking treatment for wrist or hand pain, however, about 20 percent have hypermobility, a condition that can lead to increased stress on joints, causing pain in the fingers and wrist.

Gender

Many studies show that female musicians experience a higher incidence of medical problems than their male counterparts. The reasons for this are not entirely clear. We do know that women tend to seek healthcare in general sooner than men, and that may be why they are over-represented in surveys of musicians. Women also tend to have smaller muscles and are less likely to engage in activities that maintain upper body and arm strength. The potential for mismatch between player and instrument size may also be a factor. For example, plucking the strings on the harp requires much more force than playing other string instruments, yet it is almost an exclusively female pursuit.

Quality of Instrument

While not all musicians can afford top-quality instruments, maintaining the instrument they have is important. Woodwind and brass instruments with sticky or leaky valves can increase stress on fingers and tendons. Similarly, a stringed instrument with a bridge that is too high, or a piano with worn felt, can require extra force that increases the risk of injury.

Environmental Factors

Performing and practicing in poorly lit and chilly environments such as outdoor festivals or cold basement practice rooms can also lead to injuries. At low temperatures, nerve conduction is slowed, which may decrease your sensitivity or increase the perceived force needed to play. Joints tend to be less flexible, slowing dexterity. Dressing more warmly and undertaking a longer and more thorough warm-up can help.

RISKS ASSOCIATED WITH INSTRUMENTS

Keyboard

The speed, intricacy, difficulty, and hand stretch required to perform specific keyboard compositions, along with the repetitions, place keyboard players at risk of injury. Hand and wrist position over the keys is important, as is the keyboard itself. Arthur Rubinstein traveled with his own pianos, which were designed for especially light resistance to enhance his speed and ease of play.

Violin and Viola

Studies have shown significant differences between violinists and violists in developing overuse injuries. Violists have a higher incidence of injuries, which correlates with the larger width and length of the viola relative to that of the violin.

Cello

The need for prolonged elbow flexion when playing the cello can contribute to ulnar nerve problems. The larger, thicker, and heavier bow can lead to right hand pain with bow grip.

Double Bass

The unwieldy size of the double bass and different playing styles can contribute to a variety of problems. Classical music is typically played with a bow, and problems with the bow hand can occur as with the cello. In jazz and popular music, the strings are plucked with a motion that can lead to problems with the index finger and thumb. Excessive wrist flexion with plucking should be avoided.

Harp

The harp presents problems because of its size and weight, as well as with the required playing positions. Excessive shoulder abduction and wrist extension can lead to problems with tendonitis in these areas.

Guitar

Classical and popular styles of guitar playing vary considerably but both place strains on the hands. Excessive wrist flexion should be avoided to reduce pressure on the nerves and tendons at the wrist. The position of the forearm as it rests on the edge of the guitar body can cause localized pressure in that area, leading to pain or numbness.

Wind and Brass Instruments

Hand and arm problems from depressing keys and supporting wind or brass instruments are common. Supporting of brass and woodwind instruments with the hands can often cause pain in the thumbs.

Although this list of hazards can be alarming, there's good news, too: with proper physical conditioning and playing technique, you can enjoy a long career as a performing or amateur musician.

OVERUSE SYMPTOMS

The most common symptom of overuse or repetitive strain injuries is pain, ranging from mild discomfort to sharp shooting pain and spasms. It will help the doctor you consult if you can categorize your symptoms clearly. Consider the following list and see what describes your situation best:

- pain at one site only, and only while playing
- pain at multiple sites
- pain that persists beyond playing
- pain with and beyond playing, including pain with other nonmusical activities
- pain with and beyond playing, and whenever the affected body area is used

Other symptoms can include a "pins and needles" sensation or electric shock–like feeling more typically associated with nerve compression. Cold extremities, with reduced blood flow due to environmental temperature or spasm of arteries, can cause pain or numbness.

WHAT TO EXPECT WHEN YOU SEEK MEDICAL ATTENTION

Ask around and, if you can, find a doctor who is familiar with instrument-specific problems that can occur in professional musicians. During your first appointment with a hand specialist, the doctor should review three areas. Not surprisingly, the examination will start with a review of your medical history. Then, the doctor should perform a physical examination of you without your musical instrument, followed by (whenever possible) an examination of you playing the instrument.

History

A detailed chronological history of your symptoms can provide clues to the cause of the injury, in addition to revealing your playing routines, previous medical treatment, and general fitness and health.

Physical Examination

Although musicians often come to a hand specialist with a complaint of a hand or forearm problem on one side, the medical examination needs to include both arms as well as the back. The musician's posture should be examined, too. Manual muscle testing to detect strength deficits, including the hand's intrinsic muscles, should be made and compared to the opposite side. The doctor may also want to perform tests for nerve compression in the neck and arms. Active and passive range of motion, joint laxity, and hypermobility are also important elements of a thorough exam.

Examination with the Musical Instrument

If the doctor can examine you playing your instrument, she will glean valuable information that can help you get the best treatment. Whether seated or standing, your posture will be assessed, too, and since many musicians begin training at a young age, asymmetric physical development or physical accommodation to the instrument will be looked for. Excessive tension and excessive flexion will also be assessed. The musician can be completely unaware of the amount of wrist flexion or extension while playing, but the doctor will observe it. Violin and viola players may hyperflex the wrist when playing at the higher registers; holding the guitar too low while playing can also excessively flex the wrist; flutists may hyperextend the left wrist while playing; and so on. Improper playing technique is the culprit, not the act of musicianship itself.

COMMON DIAGNOSES

Nerve Compression Syndromes

Pressure on peripheral nerves can occur at any age and in any occupation but professional musicians are at an increased risk. The nerves to the hands are almost 3 feet long, beginning in the neck and extending to the fingertips. External pressure on a nerve leads to symptoms ranging from nonspecific aching in the hand or arm to localized pain, numbness, or tingling. Nerve compression affecting the upper extremity can originate in the neck or spine, the *thoracic outlet* (the area between the rib cage and the collar bone), elbow, or wrist.

Ulnar Nerve Entrapment

The ulnar nerve is located on the inside of the elbow in the "funny bone" area. *Ulnar nerve entrapment* symptoms include pain or discomfort at the elbow often with radiating numbness or tingling to the small finger. Weakness or loss of dexterity in the affected hand can also occur. Excessive or repetitive elbow flexion can compress the nerve, and because the muscles that flex the fingers and wrist surround the ulnar nerve, playing with excessive tension or wrist flexion can also compress it.

Carpal Tunnel Syndrome

The *median nerve* is the other main nerve that provides feeling in the hand. It controls muscles and feeling to the thumb, index finger, middle finger, and thumb side of the ring finger. (The little finger side of the ring finger and the little finger are supplied by the *ulnar nerve*, as noted above.) There is a "tunnel" at the wrist that the median nerve passes through. Excessive wrist flexion or extension can increase pressure within the carpal tunnel and can contribute to the development of *carpal tunnel syndrome*, causing numbness and tingling in the wrist and in the fingers. (Carpal tunnel syndrome is covered in chapter 9.)

Musculoskeletal Pain and Overuse Syndromes

By far the most common reason that performing artists and musicians seek medical attention is for muscle and tendon problems. Musicians can develop common tendon inflammations like *de Quervain tendonitis* of the thumb, medial and lateral *epicondylitis* of the elbow, and *stenosing tenosynovitis*, or "trigger finger," in the hand. These problems usually respond well to treatment.

It may surprise you to learn from your doctor that muscle weakness in the upper extremity, shoulder, and core trunk muscles can lead to excessive tension and pain in the hand and forearm. Gentle exercises can be combined with a more general upper body conditioning program. Treatment by a physical or occupational therapist familiar with musicians, combined with Alexander or Feldenkrais method therapy to minimize excessive tension in muscles, has proven very successful.

Focal Dystonia

Focal dystonia, also known as occupational cramp or "writer's cramp," remains a poorly understood condition characterized by involuntary loss of fine muscle control. It usually is noted as a painless loss of muscle control during a particular skilled movement such as playing a musical instrument. Although the cause remains unknown, some believe that repetition of highly complex coordinated motions for a prolonged period of time can "damage" the specific nerves required for that specific motion. Musicians with focal dystonia may only have difficulty when playing their instruments while other tasks, such as typing, can be unaffected.

Focal dystonia usually develops during or after an intense or prolonged practice of a difficult or new passage, when attempting to learn a new technique, or when changing an instrument. Typically, the small and ring fingers are more involved, but in banjo and guitar players the index and middle fingers can be involved. Whatever digit is affected, the finger tends to curl or straighten involuntarily. Although this problem is rare, it has affected some famous musicians. In recent times, well-known pianists have had to alter their careers because of focal dystonia. Leon Fleisher was one (figure 5.1).

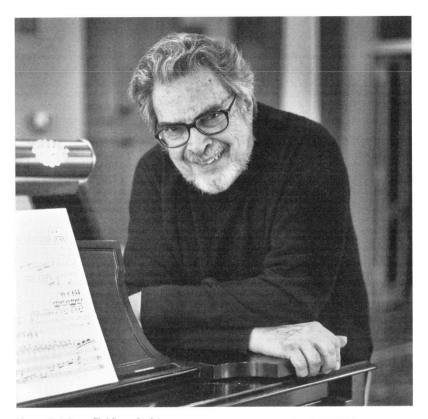

Figure 5.1. Leon Fleisher, pianist. COURTESY LEON FLEISHER AND CHRIS HARTLOVE

Fleisher sought many medical opinions and treatments for his focal dystonia, but nothing provided relief. He became deeply depressed when he could no longer perform, and eventually turned to teaching. When he discovered the works for the left-hand-only (commissioned by Paul Wittgenstein, a wealthy Viennese pianist who lost his right arm in World War I), he resumed some concert playing. With the use of *Botox (botulinum toxin, a medicine made from a bacteria, which when injected into muscles, temporarily paralyses or weakens them)* to weaken the spastic muscles in his right hand, combined with *Rolfing* (a deep tissue massage technique), he was able to regain some use of his right hand, and in 1995 gave a two-handed performance with the Cleveland Orchestra and is still performing and teaching.

RETURN TO PLAY

Treating performing musicians is similar to treating professional athletes: the first step is to diagnose and treat the source of the pain, and the second is returning the musician to the stage. Because of the emotional stress caused by being away from their instruments, musicians are often tempted to leap back into playing as soon as they start to improve, but true healing requires a gradual and methodical plan to begin and increase playing time. An incomplete recovery only sets the stage for further injury. You, your doctor, and your therapists should work together to create a back-to-play schedule to minimize the urge to advance too quickly.

Although there are no studies on the ideal return-to-play schedule, many find that a schedule divided into play and rest periods gives the best results. Playing times should never extend to the point where pain occurs. Breaking practice time into 1-hour blocks is usually helpful, and each session should begin with a 5- to 10-minute warm-up using the large muscle groups. After the warm-up, a period of play, usually lasting 5 minutes, follows. The next step is a cool-down period, away from the instrument. The remaining time in the hour should be rest.

At first a single cycle per day may be all you can handle, but as healing progresses the cycle can be repeated more than once a day. When 2 or 3 cycles can be done without pain, the playing time can be increased in 3- to 5-minute increments every 3 to 7 days as long as you are not experiencing pain. Your ultimate goal is a 1-hour practice schedule consisting of a 10-minute warm-up, 40 minutes of playing, and a 10-minute cool-down period—all without pain.

The story of the race between the tortoise and the hare that we all learned as children is true when it comes to healing and rehabilitation: "Slow and steady wins the race."

CHAPTER 6

I SEE WHAT YOU MEAN

◆

*Hearing with Your Eyes and Speaking with
Your Hands in American Sign Language*

Rebecca J. Saunders, P.T., C.H.T.

Grace Benham was born deaf. But that wasn't the only challenge she faced; she also had a heart defect and a cyst at the base of her spine that made it difficult for her to stand or walk. But as a deaf child, Grace had another pressing problem: *radial aplasia*, a congenital condition that meant she had no thumb on her right hand and no radius (one of the two bones that runs from the wrist to the elbow). Without fully functioning hands, it would be difficult for Grace to communicate.

Fortunately for Grace, she was adopted by a couple who did not view her medical problems, including her deafness, as significant obstacles to leading a full life. As a matter of fact, her adoptive mother, Nancy Benham, Ph.D., worked at a school for the deaf. She believed strongly that there is "nothing wrong with being deaf." She knew that Grace would acquire language. As Dr. Benham pointed out, "We use that language at home." She was referring to American Sign Language (ASL).

Grace's heart defect was corrected when she was 6 months old and the cyst on her spine was removed when she was 2. The problem of not having a thumb, however, remained. Because many of the words and letters used in ASL require a thumb, the lack of one meant Grace could not "speak" with her parents—or with anyone else, for that matter.

The Benhams had heard there were hand surgeons who could re-shape a hand and provide a thumb by moving the index finger to the thumb position. This procedure is known as a pollicization (as described in chapter 2). Eventually, the Benhams were referred to Dr. Mark Baratz, an orthopedic hand specialist at Allegheny General Hospital in Pittsburgh, Pennsylvania.

Dr. Baratz, who had studied sign language when he was a medical student, first saw Grace and her parents in September 2005. "I had done lots of different operations to rebuild the thumb, to realign the thumb," Dr. Baratz said. "It's one of the more common things that we do on children. But [Grace's case] was the first time that I did an operation on a child who couldn't speak, couldn't hear, and needed this hand not only for eating, playing, and working, but also for communicating," he noted. "So for me, the stakes were higher."

After discussing the surgical alternatives with the Benhams, the decision was made to go with the pollicization procedure. The index finger on Grace's right hand would be surgically manipulated to become her new thumb, leaving her with three fingers on her right hand rather than four. Although Grace's right hand was always in a cast or splint for about a year after her surgery, it didn't slow her down. She continued to play, learn, and express a desire to be doing what everybody else was doing. Grace's parents, her doctor, and her teachers agreed: the surgery had been a success.

Eventually, Grace's remarkable story made the news. In 2007, Dan Majors of the *Pittsburgh Post-Gazette* reported on the little girl's journey to acquire a new language, captivating readers with the resilience of the 4-year-old child who had started life with so many challenges. One of the interviews included Mary Ann Stefko, a coordinator at the school Grace attended. Describing the change she saw in Grace, Stefko said, "At first, she was very quiet, very cautious, and very reluctant to sign. What I've seen since she's been here is the total blossoming of a little girl. It really is like watching a bloom open up."

Grace became "more and more enthusiastic about signing" and more willing to use both hands. It wasn't long before she was acquiring ASL even faster than her peers. She was, as Ms. Stefko pointed out, "probably a little bit ahead of a typical 4-year-old."

In the United States today, there are nearly 29 million deaf individuals. Deafness is a medical condition, but it's more than that. It also imparts a cultural identity. The deaf are a sociolinguistic minority with their own traditions, interests, and behaviors. There is a unique deaf language—sign language, a way of communicating that requires the use of the hands (figure 6.1).

Degrees and types of deafness vary. Two common terms used to refer to individuals in the deaf community are *deaf* and *hard of hearing*. (The term *hearing impaired* is not favored by the deaf community because they do not believe deafness is a disability.) Most deaf individuals have some residual hearing; those without any residual hearing are considered severely and profoundly deaf. As you may know from your own family or circle of friends, deaf individuals can use hearing aids to amplify environmental sounds. Hearing aids, however, do not allow a deaf person to hear speech. Fully functional hands, therefore, are extremely important to the deaf, as they supply the primary means of communication.

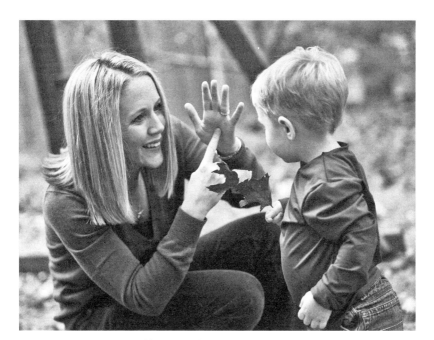

Figure 6.1. Signing the word leaf using the ASL alphabet

In their book, *Deaf in America: Voices from a Culture*, Carol Padden and Tom Humphries explain the difference between the terms *deaf* and *Deaf*. The lowercase *deaf* refers to the audiological condition of not hearing, whereas the uppercase *Deaf* refers to a group of deaf people who share culture and a language, ASL.

Deafness also is categorized based on when the hearing loss occurred. A person is described as pre-lingually or post-lingually deaf, or late-deafened. *Pre-lingually deaf* means the person was deaf before the acquisition of language; *post-lingually deaf* means the deafness occurred after language acquisition. *Late-deafened* refers to individuals who lost hearing at a later stage of life. Why any of this matters is that the person's age at the onset of deafness affects which mode of communication he will use as the primary method.

Although only 10 percent of deaf children are born to deaf parents, early exposure to sign language allows them to learn ASL as their primary language and helps them learn English. Studies of the recent trend to teach infants "baby sign" have shown that it can accelerate language development and decrease frustrations in communication for both the child and parents. Prelingually deaf children can begin to learn sign language as early as 6 to 8 months of age. Teaching usually begins with three to five signs and, because speech remains a goal, words are usually used along with the signs. Eye contact and emphasis on the word also help to convey meaning.

For a person to become fluent in any language, exposure needs to begin early, preferably before school age. For those learning ASL, whether it will be a first or second language, age is a critical issue. Native signers (those born deaf who learned ASL in infancy) consistently display more accomplished sign ability than non-native signers. This difference emphasizes the importance of early exposure to and acquisition of ASL and thus, the vital need for hand and finger dexterity.

HISTORY OF DEAF EDUCATION AND
AMERICAN SIGN LANGUAGE

Born and raised in France, Laurent Clerc came to the United States in 1816 and within a year became the first deaf teacher of the deaf in America; because of his significant work with and accomplishments for the deaf, he is referred to as "the apostle of the deaf in America." As co-founder of the first American school for the deaf in 1817 in Hartford, Connecticut (originally called the American Asylum at Hartford for the Education and Instruction of the Deaf and Dumb, now the American School for the Deaf), Clerc was the first proponent in the United States of sign language instruction over oral instruction. His understanding of the Deaf's natural inclination to use sign language formed the basis of his view of deafness as a minority culture, similar to other language minority groups that exist in the middle of a major culture.

Edward Minor Gallaudet, a friend of Clerc and a fellow-Frenchman and advocate for sign language, was a teacher at Clerc's Hartford school. In 1857, Gallaudet became superintendent at the Columbia Institution for the Deaf and Dumb in Washington, D.C. In 1864, the U.S. Congress passed an act, signed by Abraham Lincoln, making it the National Deaf-Mute College, which later achieved university status and was renamed Gallaudet University.

Although there are more than 100 different sign languages in use around the world, ASL is unique as a visual language in that it uses manual signs, body language, and facial expressions to convey meaning. It is the predominant sign language of Deaf Americans, which includes the Deaf communities of English-speaking parts of Canada. Distinct from spoken English, ASL has its own semantics, syntax, and grammar. After English and Spanish, ASL is the third most commonly used language in the United States.

When performing ASL, the person signing expresses information through combinations of hand shapes, palm orientations, placement of the hand in space in relation to the body, movement of the body, and facial expressions (figure 6.2). For instance, a question is indicated by raising the eyebrows and widening the eyes or by leaning forward and using these facial expressions. Most of the information conveyed is by

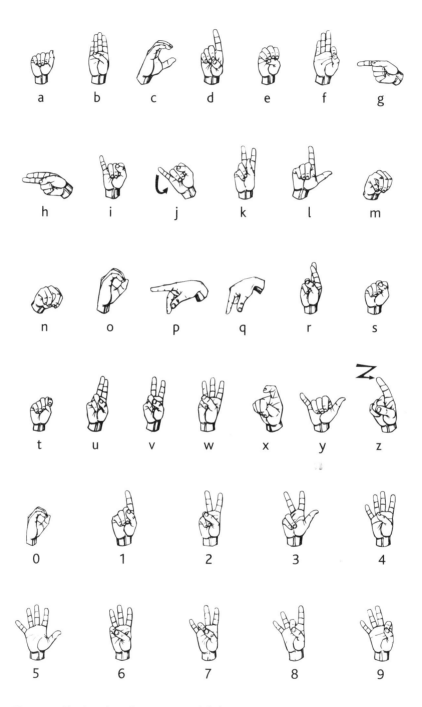

Figure 6.2. The American Sign Language alphabet.

the dominant hand while the non-dominant hand serves as a base or as a mirror image.

So, you can imagine how serious it is for an ASL-user to lose the use of the dominant hand; if that happens, signing becomes as difficult as learning to write with your non-dominant hand, a task that increases in difficulty the older you are. If you have ever fractured the wrist or arm of your dominant hand, you know exactly how awkward and arduous it is to learn to use the other hand for writing.

Finger-spelling is another form of sign language. It uses different finger positions to spell out letters of the alphabet and to convey numbers. Finger-spelling is part of ASL, used primarily for proper nouns, emphasis, clarity, and instruction.

Signed English is another type of manual communication. It differs from ASL by putting signs in spoken English word order, a sequence not used in ASL. Signed English is considered cumbersome and imposes a strain on those who use it. The linguistic researcher Ursula Bellugi reported that deaf people said they could process each item as it appeared but found it difficult to process the message content as a whole. This difficulty is due to neurological limitations in normal short-term memory and cognitive processing. Another researcher, Sam Supalla, found that deaf children exposed only to Signed English "replace its grammatical devices with purely spatial ones similar to those found in ASL or other signed languages." All indigenous sign languages have very similar spatial structure, and they do not resemble Signed English or signed speech, which is why it's not surprising that wherever there are groups of deaf people, signed languages evolve separately and independently from spoken language.

RECOGNITION OF DEAFNESS

A *hearing impairment*, or *deafness*, is a partial or full decrease in the ability to detect or process sounds. Fifty percent of congenital hearing impairments have no known cause but there are some known prenatal risk factors, including rubella, CMV (*cytomegalovirus*, the most common viral infection in fetuses and a leading cause of deafness), and other infectious diseases (toxoplasmosis, herpes, syphilis, and flu among them). Consumption of illicit drugs and/or alcohol by a pregnant woman as well as *ototoxic drugs* (medicines that can damage hearing) have also been linked to deafness.

Symptoms of congenital deafness in newborns include:

- lack of response to loud noise
- lack of response to voices or noise when sleeping in a quiet room
- failure to calm down in response to the mother's voice
- failure to make normal baby sounds like cooing by 6 weeks of age
- failure to look for the source of a noise by 3 to 6 months of age
- failure to play with noisy toys by 6 to 8 months of age
- failure to babble by about 6 months of age

Symptoms that a baby or young child has a hearing impairment include:

- lack of reaction to loud noises
- failure to imitate sounds
- lack of response to her name during the first year of life
- failure to vocalize (imitating sounds, playing games that involve speech, or
- talking in two-word sentences) by the age of 2
- failure to understand simple directions by the third year

Parents are usually the first to suspect their child has a hearing impairment; when this is a concern, the pediatrician should be contacted immediately. Early detection and intervention for hearing impairments is crucial in order to prevent or minimize developmental and educational delays. Studies have shown that hearing-impaired children who are identified and receive intervention before 6 months of age develop significantly better language skills than children who are identified after 6 months of age. Many hearing-impaired and deaf infants who are signed to from birth begin to use baby signs by as early as 7 months of age.

In the United States, the average age of diagnosis of hearing loss is at about 2 years old, but studies show significant hearing impairments have gone undiagnosed in children as old as 6. Early diagnosis of a child who is deaf or hard of hearing is crucial to ensure that the family has the resources they need to help the child acquire language, visual and/or spoken. It also helps the child reach appropriate communicative, cognitive, academic, social, and emotional development. For this reason, the National Association of the Deaf (NAD) supported passage of the Early Hearing Detection and Intervention Act (EHDI) in 2000. The goals of the EHDI program includes screening of all newborns by 1 month of age, confirmation of their hearing status by 3 months of age, and enrollment in early intervention programs for deaf and hard of hearing babies and their families by 6 months of age.

The NAD states that acquiring language from birth is a human right. It supports the concept that deaf and hard of hearing infants should be given the opportunity to acquire ASL as early as possible in addition to the opportunity to access and acquire the spoken language(s) used by their families.

THE STRESS ON HANDS OF THE DEAF

Dr. Roy Meals, an orthopedic hand surgeon from the UCLA Medical Center, did a study on the functional demands and consequences of manual communication. He and his colleagues studied 15 deaf signers with upper limb abnormalities, aged 5 to 83 years, to determine how their abnormalities affected their signing. They also looked at overuse syndromes in 6 sign language interpreters. Of the 21 individuals studied, 9 had stiff or missing digits as a result of an injury. Other problems included trigger thumb, Dupuytren contracture, and an ischemic and painful small finger. The researchers found that these impairments resulted in looser signing patterns but minimal loss of content; think of it as reading someone's poor handwriting or listening to a person with a foreign accent or mild vocal impairment.

Two of the deaf people in Dr. Meals's study had congenital limb deficiencies. One person had bilateral *radial aplasia*: no thumb on one side and a hypoplastic thumb (small and not fully functional) on the other. His signing was severely affected by the combined problems of a lack of forearm rotation and wrist extension as well as supple finger movement. The other individual had bilateral *ulnar dimelia* (she had no thumbs and was missing one of the forearm bones, on both sides, creating an unusual posture of the hand). One of her hands had six digits and the other had five. Both of her forearms were fixed in slight *pronation* (palms facing downward). At 5 years of age she had been evaluated for thumb reconstruction. At the time, her signing was severely impaired and she could only communicate effectively with close family members who were accustomed to her unique sign patterns. She underwent bilateral *pollicization* (transfer of the index finger to provide a thumb) and her ability to sign improved greatly, although the lack of forearm rotation still required a looser formation of some signs.

The upper limb problems of the six sign language interpreters included some common overuse inflammation symptoms: shoulder bursitis, *flexor tenosynovitis* ("trigger finger"), *lateral epicondylitis* ("tennis elbow"), radial tunnel syndrome, and carpal tunnel syndrome. These problems are exacerbated by interpreting in classroom and public speaking settings for lengthy periods without adequate breaks. Signing for a person who is both blind and deaf adds another degree of difficulty; in these instances, the deaf person rests her hands on top of the interpreter's in order to feel the communication. Signing against the resistance of someone's overlying hands can be exhausting for the upper extremity even when it is only done for short periods. Hand surgeons and certified hand therapists can help address these problems and therefore play an important role in the lives of the deaf and those who use sign language to communicate.

◆

With the use of ASL, countless deaf individuals are leading happy, productive lives, and are fully engaged with the hearing and non-hearing world. A contemporary list of famous Americans whose accomplishments span all areas of human endeavor includes an impressive representation of the deaf. From acting to writing, teaching to professional sports, and the arts to the media, the deaf are leaving a mark. And it all started with their hands.

CHAPTER 7

LIFE IS WHAT HAPPENS WHEN YOU'RE BUSY MAKING OTHER PLANS

◆

Injuries at Work and at Home

Keith A. Segalman, M.D.

In 1833, the Scottish anatomist Sir Charles Bell published *The Hand: Its Mechanism and Vital Endowments as Evincing Design*. His description of the human hand reads more like a love letter than a medical text, calling the hand "so beautifully formed, it has so fine sensibility, that sensibility governs its motion so correctly, every effort of the will is answered so instantly, as if the hand itself were the seat of that will; its actions are powerful, so free, and yet so delicate, that it seems to possess a quality instinct in itself, and there is no thought of its complexity as an instrument, or of the relations which make it subservient to the mind: we use it as we draw our breath, unconsciously." Clearly, he was enthralled by the amazingly exquisite nature of the hand, and rightly so.

Even if you've never pondered the hand to the degree that Sir Bell did, you can, no doubt, think of endless ways it is essential to your daily life. Any injury to the hand, therefore, can be devastating. If the bones are broken, the hand is out of commission for weeks; then, there's the worry about permanent deformities. If the nerves are injured, sensation is damaged; will it ever be restored? If the skin is cut, there's pain and the chance of infection and, possibly, an unsightly permanent scar. If the circulation is altered in a traumatic injury, will there be enough blood flow to allow normal function of the hand, particularly in the cold?

Although we all want to avoid injuries of any kind, bad things can happen to good people. But it's possible to lead a productive life even if you have severe injuries to your hand. As the many examples in this book demonstrate, people from all walks of life who have injured hands continue on to successful careers and happy lives.

Donald K. "Deke" Slaton, who lost part of a finger in a childhood farm accident, went on to become an air force pilot and later an astronaut on the *Apollo-Soyez* mission in the 1970s. Boris Yeltsin, president of the Soviet Union from 1988 to 1999, lost two of his fingers when playing with a grenade as a boy.

Mordicai Brown, an American Major League Baseball player from 1903 to 1916, had only three fingers on his dominant hand (and none of them were in very good shape). His hand had been severely mangled in a threshing machine accident when he was a child, and while he was recovering from that trauma he injured his hand again in a fall, leaving two fingers permanently paralyzed. Yet, Brown learned to play baseball and eventually became a successful pitcher known for his curve ball.

Django Reinhart became a renowned gypsy jazz guitarist with an international following in the mid-twentieth century despite the fact that two fingers on his left hand had been badly burned in a fire when he was 18. Although the fingers remained partially paralyzed, he taught himself to play the guitar in a new way, using his two healthy fingers to play melody and the injured fingers only for chord work.

All of these individuals, along with those highlighted in other chapters of this book, show that people who sustain traumatic hand injuries—even those that result in loss of digits or deformity—not only can overcome the problem but can excel in their chosen fields.

HAND INJURIES

Every year, hand injuries account for nearly 10 percent of all visits to hospital emergency rooms. The most frequent injuries are *lacerations* (cuts), *contusions* (bruises), *fractures* (broken bones), and *infections*.

Most work, whether we are engaged in a white-collar profession or blue-collar industry, requires the use of our hands. Although many workers in America have moved away from manual labor compared to those in past generations, even computer use requires dexterity, mobility, and sensibility. The jobs that we refer to as "just requiring a good brain"—research, teaching, writing, and so on—require the use of our hands as well. A hand injury is, at the very least, an impediment in any of these occupations. Untreated, a hand injury can impair function, cause chronic pain, and prevent gainful employment.

The hand and wrist consist of 27 bones and a variety of nerves, arteries, veins, muscles, tendons, and ligaments (see figure 1.1). Because of the hand's intricate anatomy, even injuries that appear to be minor have the potential to develop into serious handicaps, which is why prompt and appropriate treatment is essential and can prevent long-term disability. Virtually any injury to the hand should elicit a rapid response for first aid, and any serious injury needs to be evaluated by a hand specialist as soon as possible.

HAND INJURY SYMPTOMS AND HOME CARE

The symptoms of hand injuries vary depending on the type of injury; how the injury occurred; and the depth, severity, and location of the injury. The most common injuries are lacerations, fractures, soft tissue injuries and amputations, infections, and burns. Simple first-aid techniques can be used at home to care for most hand injuries initially, but any serious injury requires evaluation and treatment from a hand surgeon immediately. Act fast when there is:

- uncontrolled bleeding
- numbness in the digits
- pain that is uncontrolled with rest, elevation, and ice
- obvious deformity or amputation
- any of the signs of infection, such as tenderness, local warmth, redness, swelling, purulent drainage (pus), or fever

- exposure of any underlying structures, such as tendons, bones, joints, arteries, or nerves
- burns that have disrupted the skin or extend circumferentially around the finger, hand, or wrist

Lacerations (Cuts)

Lacerations can cause tenderness, pain, bleeding, numbness, decreased range of motion, stiffness, weakness, and *pallor* (a pale or bloodless appearance). To treat a laceration at home, follow these steps:

- Apply pressure to the wound to stop the bleeding.
- Elevate the hand above the heart.
- Gently wash dirt or debris from the wound with mild soap and water.
- Cover the wound to prevent further contamination (sterile gauze is ideal but any clean bandage is sufficient).
- Do not remove large foreign bodies such as nails, hooks, or knives; let the doctor do that.
- Lacerations longer than a half inch are best treated with *sutures* (stitches), which a doctor should do.

Fractures (Broken Bones) and Dislocations

Fractures and dislocations cause tenderness, deformity, swelling and discoloration, decreased range of motion, and sometimes bleeding. To treat a suspected fracture:

- Immobilize or splint the hand with whatever is available—even a piece of wood or cardboard with tape can help.
- If the bone is exposed (*open or compound fracture*), wash the wound with water and cover it with a clean bandage.
- Ice will help decrease the pain.
- Contact a hand surgeon or go to the closest emergency room.

Soft Tissue Injuries and Amputations

Soft tissue injuries and amputations are serious. Start by calling 911. Then:

- Apply pressure to the wound to stop bleeding.
- Elevate the hand above the heart.
- Gently wash dirt or debris from the wound with mild soap and water.
- Cover the wound to prevent further contamination (sterile gauze is ideal but any clean bandage is sufficient).
- Retrieve the amputated body part, keep it damp, and place it near but not on ice to keep it cool (do not the place body part in direct contact with ice because that will damage the tissue).

Infections

Hand infections that warrant medical attention include any in which there is excessive tenderness and/or warmth, redness, swelling, fever, deformity, and decreased range of motion. In those instances:

- Keep the area clean and dry.
- Elevate the hand above the heart.
- See a hand surgeon as soon as possible.

Burns

Burns can be mild or severe causing blistering, loss of tissue, redness, discoloration, tenderness, or complete numbness. Here are the first steps to follow:

- For a thermal (heat) burn: cool with water, not ice, and then cover. Never cover burns on your skin with butter or grease.
- For a chemical burn: irrigate with large amounts of water.
- For frostbite: rapidly warm by soaking in a warm-water bath.
- ALWAYS see a hand surgeon as soon as possible with any serious burn.

WHEN TO SEEK MEDICAL CARE

In many instances you can and should immediately treat a hand injury that occurs at home (or work), even if you will be also seeking medical attention as quickly as possible.

Lacerations (Cuts) and Bruises

Unless the cut occurs around or right above the wrist, it is rare that the bleeding cannot be controlled with pressure to the wound and elevation of the hand/arm. If the laceration is longer than a half inch, it will need to be sutured by a doctor. In any laceration injury, infection is always a concern; adequate cleansing is important. For sharp lacerations, such as those from a knife, gentle washing with soap and water is the best antiseptic and can be done at home. Iodine-based liquids, such as beta-dine, have not been shown to be superior to ordinary household soap and water. Alcohol-based cleaners will cause severe burning. When soap and water are not available, peroxide is an excellent alternative and will not cause burning. If there is foreign material in the wound, it needs to be removed to minimize the risk of infection. Necrotic skin should be *debrided* (removed). It is difficult for an emergency room physician to make decisions on the extent of the debridement required, which is why it is best to have a hand surgeon evaluate the injury.

In cases where there is extensive skin loss from the injury, such as the kind of abrasion that can occur when an arm is hanging out of the window during a motor vehicle accident, the expertise of a hand surgeon is essential. It may be necessary to graft skin or perform flap coverage of the wound. (For details of this procedure, see the discussion of mutilating work-related injuries later in this chapter.)

When a hand surgeon evaluates a laceration, she focuses on the potential injury to nerves, blood vessels, or tendons that has been sustained. Though treatment of injuries to these vital structures can occasionally be delayed, there is a specific window of opportunity after which repair will no longer be possible. Emergency room physicians are well qualified in their specialty—emergency medicine—but they do not have the expertise to make a decision about whether hand surgery is required. Be sure to ask that a hand surgeon evaluate your injury. (I have treated too many injuries for which inaccurate information was given by the emergency room physician, resulting in an unfortunate delay in treatment.) Oftentimes, delay means that reconstruction rather than repair will be the only option, which means full function of the hand will be compromised.

Bruises occur because of bleeding beneath the skin (*hematoma* is the medical term for *bruise*). These are not life threatening and it is rare that a hematoma needs to be treated, although many patients are bothered by the appearance of the hematoma. Most hematomas are treated by ice, elevation, and, sometimes, splinting. There are times, however, when a bruise can be a sign of an underlying fracture that may require x-rays to be correctly diagnosed.

The surgical approach to a simple laceration of the hand includes:

- anesthetizing the area, usually with local anesthesia
- cleansing and irrigating the wound
- debridement (removal) of necrotic (dead) tissue
- wound repair or closure
- dressing and splinting, if necessary, to keep hand from moving
- pain medication as needed
- tetanus shot, if necessary

Simple lacerations do not routinely require antibiotics unless the injury is the result of an animal or human bite.

Bites

Bites can be inflicted by animals (usually dogs and cats) or by people. The main complication of bite wounds is infection. To help prevent infection, bite wounds require thorough cleansing and *irrigation* (washing) of the wound. Puncture wounds (such as cat bites) and wounds where tissue is crushed (such as human and dog bites) are particularly likely to become infected. The risk of infection increases when these wounds are sutured, so bite wounds almost always need to be allowed to heal without stitches. Most bite wounds will require antibiotics and close follow-up to assure healing.

One of the more common causes of a human bite wound is a fight in which a punch results in a cut when the hand strikes the opponent's teeth. When this kind of "fight bite" is located over a joint (usually the knuckle), it may be necessary to clean the joint in a way that can only be done properly in the operating room. It is rare for animal bites to cause a fracture (broken bone) but it is not unusual for a human bite to cause an injury to the joint surface. Be warned: this type of injury may appear minor but can lead to severe deformity or disability if not appropriately treated. Unfortunately, many patients with a human bite injury do not seek early treatment—when the prognosis for recovery is excellent—and only come to the emergency room when an established infection is present.

Tendon Injuries

The hand has an intricate arrangement of flexor and extensor tendons (see figure 1.1). Although most fingers have two flexor tendons, a laceration of the deep (profundus) flexor tendon will result in an inability to bring a finger into the palm (to make a fist). Many people will resist moving a finger after a laceration because of the pain, but true inability to move the finger requires the evaluation of a hand surgeon. For optimal outcome, flexor tendon injuries require surgical repair within 7 to 10 days.

A laceration of the extensor tendon is immediately obvious because the person cannot fully extend the finger. Weakness and pain when attempting to extend the digits should be evaluated by a hand surgeon. I do not recommend relying on an emergency room physician's opinion that "everything is okay" if symptoms persist after a laceration. Extensor tendon lacerations require surgical repair.

The most common type of extensor tendon injury is not a laceration but a mallet injury ("baseball finger"). The tip of the digit is jammed and forced into flexion. The terminal extensor tendon is pulled from its attachment at the end of the bone, making it impossible for the person to extend the terminal portion of the digit. These injuries rarely require surgery but are frustrating to treat. Mallet deformities require full-time, not-ever-to-be-removed (until treatment is complete) splinting of the tip of the finger for 8 weeks. The condition improves but often is never fully corrected.

Dislocations and Fractures

A *dislocation* occurs when a joint is displaced out of its normal position and results in obvious deformity, pain, and a decrease in mobility. When a dislocation occurs, the doctor will evaluate the injury to ensure there are no fractures or bone breaks. Dislocations result from injuries to the ligaments around joints (see figure 1.1 A and B). A ligament is a supporting structure that attaches the bones together to provide stability and mobility. The joint is put back into position in a process called a *reduction*. Reduction can be accomplished by external manipulation of the injured area (*closed reduction*) or by surgery (*open reduction*). All reductions require follow-up medical care after a period of immobilization, usually with a splint or cast. The goal of the treatment is to preserve the function, regain stability of the joint, and prevent arthritis.

A closed reduction requires anesthetizing the finger and gently manipulating the joint. The joint should come back into position fairly easily. The physician should make sure the joint is stable after the reduction and obtain x-rays to confirm the joint is well-aligned. Multiple attempts at reduction are usually not helpful. If the joint cannot be manually reduced, it usually means a structure like the extensor tendon is entrapped in the joint and surgery will be required to correct the problem. There is a rare group of dislocations, including wrist and middle finger joint (proximal interphalangeal joint), dislocations that remain unstable even after an open reduction because of extensive ligament damage. These injuries usually require complex surgery to maintain joint stability. After the reduction is accomplished, the finger is usually splinted for several days to allow swelling to reduce. The greatest long-term difficulty for most dislocations is stiffness. Therefore, it is necessary to start moving the finger early on. Occasionally, two fingers are taped together for several weeks, called *buddy taping*, to provide stability (see figure 3.3). In the rare instance that the joint re-dislocates, surgery is usually necessary.

After a dislocation, many people will have permanent stiffness, and hand therapy may be required to regain function. Swelling in the joint usually persists for 3 to 6 months after a dislocation.

Fractures (broken bones) of the hand and wrist are usually accompanied by pain, deformity, swelling, and limited motion—no surprise there. No two fractures are the same, however, and the treatment will depend on a number of factors, including the location of the fracture, the amount of *displacement* (shift in the bones), whether the joint surface is involved, and if a *laceration* (cut) is associated with the fracture.

A fracture that is not displaced usually only requires protection in a splint or a cast. It is best to splint the fracture (half cast) and, after several days, place a circumferential cast (full cast). This sequence is followed because a splint allows room for the swelling associated with acute injuries, and is also intended to prevent the loss of adequate circulation or nerve injury. That said, splinting does not entirely eliminate the possibility of these complications. Anyone who experiences numbness, color change, or the feeling of tightness after splinting or casting should return to the doctor as quickly as possible.

Displaced fractures in adults generally do not respond well to closed reduction (manipulation of the fracture) and therefore require surgical intervention. Fractures that involve the joint surface almost always require surgery. During surgery, the fracture can be treated in one of two ways: it can be manipulated (the surgeon pushes on the skin and forces the fracture into position, and then places pins without making an incision), or an open reduction can be performed (an incision through the skin is made, the fracture is placed into position, and screws and plates are placed to stabilize the fracture).

Children's bones are still growing and they are susceptible to fractures through the growth plate. The *growth plate* is located near the joint and is the location where the longitudinal growth (length) occurs. Some of these growth plate injuries are difficult to diagnose because they do not show up on x-rays. Displaced fractures that involve the growth plate must be reduced surgically to prevent future growth disturbance. Growth disturbance can present itself as either angulatory growth (the finger grows crooked) or failure to grow, resulting in a shorter bone.

Amputations

Loss of fingers or the thumb (*amputations*) can cause major functional loss to the hand. Reattaching of digits (*replantation*) is difficult and, even if successful, will not result in normal hand function. Even after a successful replant, the person will still experience some permanent numbness, cold sensitivity, and stiffness. Replantation is successful about 85 percent of the time. The surgeon may be more inclined to attempt replantation when an amputation involves a child, or when the thumb is the digit that has been lost, or if there has been an amputation of several fingers or the entire hand. It is not technically possible to reattach a finger that is amputated beyond the base of the nail (fingertip). Replantation for the fingertip is controversial because the functional result is not always good enough to justify the inherent risks of surgery to the patient. The ultimate functional result of replantation of a finger usually depends on the level at which the amputation occurs. For instance, replantations of amputations between the PIP and the DIP joints, between the two knuckle joints, usually do well. Amputations where the finger meets the hand usually result in a stiff finger. The surgeon must have a discussion with the patient about the usefulness of performing this complicated and time-consuming operation. A replantation of the thumb at any level usually gives a useful result.

The method of injury is a major factor in determining whether replantation will be successful. Crushing or tearing injuries tend to injure vital structures (arteries, veins, nerves, and tendons) over a larger area than where the skin is lacerated, the so-called *zone of injury*. A large zone of injury means that grafting of injured structures will be needed, which reduces the success of surgery. For persons who smoke, there is a much lower chance that replantation will succeed because capillary growth is compromised by smoking. If an amputated part is handled properly, replantation can be successful up to 24 hours after the injury. If the amputated part is not properly cooled, replantation is not possible after 6 hours. The recovery and time before the person can return to work are vastly different for a replantation versus a *completion of amputation* in which the damaged digit is surgically shortened. In determining whether to attempt a replantation, the injured person needs to help make the decision based on the chance of success, the nature of the injury, the person's medical status, and the demands of the patient's profession.

When an amputated hand or digit can be retrieved, it should be managed in the following fashion. If saline solution is available, place the part in gauze coated with saline. If saline is not available, wrap the part in any clean object, even a paper towel. The part should then be put in an enclosed container, plastic bag, or clean plastic food container. The container should then be placed on ice (figure 7.1). Do not place the body part in direct contact with ice; freezing will damage the tissue.

Most amputations occur distal to (beyond) the nail bed and are not amenable to replantation. Amputations at the very tip of the finger without an exposed bone can be treated with dressing changes. Amputations with a large area of skin loss but no exposed bone may be skin grafted. When there is exposed bone, the options include a *revision of amputation* (closure of the wound by shortening the finger), advancing local skin, or a *cross finger graft* (webbing the adjacent fingers to rotate skin from an uninjured digit). Your hand surgeon will determine the best approach based on the nature of the injury and the amount of tissue loss.

Infection

You may be surprised to learn that infections are the most common disorder treated by hand surgeons. Fingertip and nail infections can often be treated in the doctor's office or at an emergency room with incision and drainage (if indicated), antibiotics, and close follow-up. A major consideration for an infection in the hand is fluid collection, or an *abscess*. If the infection is isolated to the skin, known as *cellulitis*, treatment involves antibiotics, splinting, and close follow-up. An abscess requires drainage (sometimes known as *lancing*). If the abscess is large or near nerves, arteries, ligaments, or tendons, it may need to be treated in the operating room. Hand infections have the potential for rapid progression leading to severe loss of function or even amputations in severe cases, so timely treatment is essential.

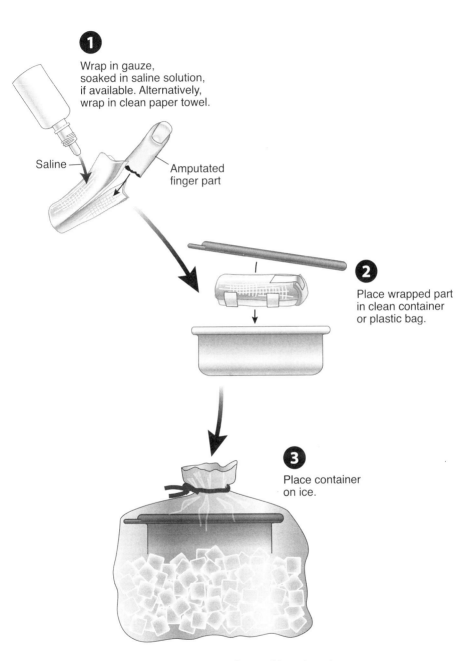

① Wrap in gauze, soaked in saline solution, if available. Alternatively, wrap in clean paper towel.

Saline

Amputated finger part

② Place wrapped part in clean container or plastic bag.

③ Place container on ice.

Figure 7.1. Preserving a severed finger part for possible replantation. ILLUSTRATION BY JACQUELINE SCHAFFER

Nerve Injuries

Nerve injuries usually occur secondary to a cut (laceration), although crush injuries can cause loss of nerve function with an intact nerve. Nerve lacerations beyond the nail plate, toward the end of the finger, usually cannot be repaired. A repair is typically done with the use of a high-powered microscope in the operating room. Unfortunately, nerves in adults do not recover completely or immediately. The nerve recovers at a rate of one inch per month; in a healthy person, 80 percent of the lost feeling will recover. If the nerve is not repaired, a *neuroma* (a painful nerve end) will result.

Burns

Serious burn injuries to the hand may require an evaluation by a hand surgeon or a burn surgeon, and hospital admission may be required for treatment. Multiple operations including skin grafting may be needed to achieve the best outcome.

A *first-degree burn* does not blister and only affects the outer layers of the skin. It should be treated with cool water. Never use salves to cool the hand for any burns! Bandaging with antibacterial ointment is sufficient. Other than discoloration of the skin, long-term complications are rare.

Second-degree burns injure the outer layers of skin and lead to blistering. They call for a visit to an emergency room. Initial treatment is to cool the injured area, which can be done by submersing the hand in cool water before you get to the emergency room. Never apply ice directly to the burn. Application of an antibacterial ointment and bandaging is the next step. A popular ointment is a sulfa-based drug called Silvadene. It is essential that during the healing process the person maintains range of motion to prevent contractures (the surrounding skin begins to tighten and pull together, which can result in restriction of movement). The wounds will heal on their own, and blisters are generally left intact until they rupture on their own.

Third-degree burns extend through the entire skin surface and may involve the tendons, nerves, and even bone. The skin is *insensate* (lacks sensation) and numb, and blisters may develop. Third-degree burns will not heal without surgery. The initial treatment is the same as for other types of burns but it is also necessary to excise the burned area and provide skin substitutes in the form of skin grafting. Occasionally, more complex types of skin flaps are required.

Chemical burns. The treatment of chemical burns depends on the chemical involved but it is usually recommended to irrigate the area with large quantities of water. If you or someone with you can do so, speak directly with your local burn center to determine the appropriate treatment. The first step involves avoiding further damage by stopping exposure to the chemical. This often means removing contaminated gloves or other clothing, and usually lots of irrigation with water. Further treatment depends on the depth of the burn. Chemical burns to the hand require specialty care from a hand surgeon or a burn center.

Electrical burns. Electrical injuries can be life-threatening because of the damage to organs such as the heart and kidneys. They should never be treated at home. The person will require cardiac monitoring for heart arrhythmias and large quantities of intravenous fluids to prevent kidney failure. The prognosis depends on the voltage exposure and the pathway of the current. The current passes along the pathway of nerves, so permanent numbness can occur. *Compartment syndrome* (swelling within a muscle compartment of the arm and leg) can lead to contracture and muscle death, artery thrombosis (a clot preventing blood flow), and even the need for amputations.

Cold Injury

Most exposure to cold causes temporary pain and little or no long-term damage. Prolonged exposure, however, can lead to tissue loss, chronic cold sensitivity, and even amputations. When hands have been exposed to cold for a long time, it is necessary to rapidly rewarm them with warm water (104° to 108°F) for 15 to 30 minutes. Sterile dressings and antibiotic creams are also required, as is care from a hand surgeon or a burn surgeon.

Blood Vessel Injuries

Blood flow enters the hand through two arteries at the wrist (the radial and ulnar arteries) that communicate with each other before sending blood to the tips of the digits. There are also two arteries in each finger that communicate with each other.

An injury or clot within one artery may be tolerated and does not always require repair or reconstruction. The decision to repair or reconstruct an arterial injury depends on the location of the injury, the time from injury to surgery, and blood flow from the other artery to the injured part of the hand or finger. If an arterial reconstruction is required, a hand surgeon will usually take a vein from the same arm or one of the legs to bridge the gap in the artery. Symptoms from the lack of adequate circulation can include ulceration at the tip of a finger, pain, numbness, and gangrene.

Blood returns from the hand to the heart through veins. Veins are either superficial (they can be seen under the skin and are used for blood drawing or intravenous lines), or they are deep in the hand and cannot be seen. Many people worry about venous injuries, but a laceration is only worrisome because it can cause bleeding. No one ever *exsanguinated* (bled out) from a superficial venous laceration, and no superficial vein ever needs to be repaired surgically.

An *aneurysm* is a dilatation (widening) in the artery, and can come from a partial injury to the vessel, *atherosclerosis* (hardening of the arteries), or repetitive pressure. The most common aneurysm is across the palm involving the ulnar artery; this is called a *hypothenar hammer syndrome*. An aneurysm causes pain and a mass, and can lead to gangrene in the fingers. An aneurysm requires surgery and can be reconstructed with a piece of vein from the arm or resected without reconstruction. The decision to reconstruct the artery depends on the back flow from the other artery and the status of the vessel above the level of the clotted area.

INJURIES AT WORK AND THEIR TREATMENT

Although all of the above mentioned injuries can occur in the workplace as well as the home, there are two others that are more commonly associated with the workplace.

Repetitive Stress

There are no medical data to confirm that repetitive activities cause overuse syndromes or resistive stress disorder. Yet, we all know that repetitive activities can lead to pain. Of the various forms of nerve compression and tendonitis, most are associated with certain demographic groups, such as postmenopausal women.

It is the job of a hand surgeon to distinguish between pain related to known diagnostic conditions, such as carpal tunnel syndrome, and other common complaints including *cubital tunnel syndrome* (compression of the ulnar "funny bone" nerve), *lateral epicondylitis* (tennis elbow), shoulder impingement (*bursitis*), and trigger finger (inflammation of the tendon sheath of the finger).

Repetitive stress disorder does not require a surgeon. Repetitive stress is treated with stretching, modification of activity, and drugs. Many individuals with repetitive stress disorder have underlying medical conditions that can predispose them to joint complaints.

Mutilating Injuries

Injuries involving multiple structures within the finger or hand are classified as *mutilating injuries*. Almost always, the injury is more extensive than it appears on initial evaluation. Medical treatment is directed to each injured structure but these injuries often have skin loss that requires more than dressing changes to get the wounds to heal. The prognosis is significantly worse when multiple systems have been injured. These types of injuries absolutely require the services of a hand surgeon; often, multiple surgeries will be necessary and full recovery can take years.

There is normally a thin covering over the tendons (the *paratenon*) to allow gliding beneath the tendon and skin. When there is extensive skin loss but the paratenon is still present, a skin graft can be used to cover the wound. The wound needs to be larger than a half inch by a half inch to even consider a skin graft. (Smaller wounds will heal on their own.) Skin grafts are either partial thickness or full thickness. A *full thickness skin graft* involves removing an area of skin (usually from the wrist or groin area), closing up the area where the skin is taken from, and placing the graft over the open area. The donor site heals with a longitudinal scar. Full thickness grafts are generally used on small areas. A *partial thickness skin graft* involves shaving a thin layer of skin, usually from the thigh, and can heal on its own. These grafts are typically used on larger areas. There are advantages and disadvantages of both types of grafts. Full thickness skin grafts usually provide more sturdy skin coverage, but partial thickness grafts have a higher success rate.

If the paratenon is missing, bone, nerve, and/or arteries are exposed, and most often a flap procedure is required. A *flap* is the placement of tissue (with circulation attached) over these vital structures (tendon, nerve, artery, or bone). Some flaps are performed by advancing (stretching) skin from local areas near the site of injury.

Pedicle flaps require other parts of the body to remain attached to the hand from distant sites such as creating "webbed" fingers (cross finger flap) or when a hand is attached to the flank (groin flap). During attachment, the skin flap will gain circulation from the injured area while still surviving on its attachment from the donor site. After 2 to 3 weeks, the hand or finger is detached and coverage is now provided for vital structures.

Some flaps are elevated, based on known patterns of circulation from the body to the skin. The most common example of this is a *radial forearm flap*. The hand surgeon will first determine that the radial artery can be sacrificed without compromising circulation to the hand. Then, skin and deeper tissue can be raised around the artery while the artery is detached from farther up the arm. The skin can now be rotated into the open area while still attached to the artery.

The final type of flap is called a *free flap*. Skin, muscle, or bone is raised from a distant site while attached to a known artery and vein.

This tissue will be placed into the defect and the artery and veins will be attached to existing ones. This requires microsurgical repair of the vessels. If muscle is transferred, the skin graft is laid over the muscle.

◆

Whether a hand injury takes place at home or at work, it is extremely important to act properly and quickly. Follow any appropriate first-aid measures that you can, and get medical attention immediately. And, if you learn that there is not a hand surgeon who can see you at the emergency room or clinic where you first seek help, ask for a referral. Your hands are worth it.

CHAPTER 8

WHEN DISEASE HURTS THE HAND

◆

Diabetes and the Hand

Kenneth R. Means Jr., M.D.

Diabetes is one of the most prevalent and serious conditions in the United States. In fact, approximately 24 million Americans have diabetes mellitus. What is perhaps more disturbing is that nearly 6 million of them are unaware they do. Ignorance is not bliss in this case; untreated diabetes leads to severely debilitating disease and complications to the entire body, including the hands.

The term *diabetes* is derived from Latin and Greek and literally means "to pass through." The word *mellitus* is Latin and means "sweetened with honey." The "honey-sweet urine" that uncontrolled diabetes causes is due to increased sugar levels in the urine. Although there are other types of diabetes, diabetes mellitus is by far the most common form of the disease. Whenever the term *diabetes* is used in this chapter, it refers to diabetes mellitus.

Diabetes is a result of the body's inability to properly use *insulin*, a hormone secreted by the pancreas, an organ located in the abdomen. Insulin is released by the pancreas whenever a person's blood sugar increases, such as after eating a meal. The insulin tells the body's cells how to use or store the sugar.

There are two basic types of diabetes. In *type 1 diabetes* (insulin-dependent diabetes), the pancreas does not produce enough insulin. In *type 2 diabetes* (insulin-resistant diabetes), the body does not use insulin properly. The end result for both types is that glucose, or sugar, levels are not properly regulated and elevated levels of sugar pass into the person's blood, urine, and body tissues.

Type 1 diabetes is most often diagnosed in childhood or adolescence. It is often characterized by a sudden and severe onset of increased blood sugar due to an insufficient production of insulin. In type 1 diabetes, the cells in the pancreas that make insulin have shut down or have been nearly completely destroyed within a very short time. The cause is unknown and is the subject of intense research. When the pancreas stops making insulin, blood sugar levels can rise to greater than five times higher than normal. These levels lead to increased urination and dehydration because the high sugar level in the blood draws fluid out from body tissues. Eventually, the person can experience loss of consciousness (*diabetic coma*) and severe fluid and electrolyte disturbances. Often, only after such a serious situation develops is the diagnosis of type 1 diabetes made.

Type 2 diabetes is the more common form and until the past 15 years or so occurred primarily in older individuals. Currently, with the epidemic of childhood and adult obesity, type 2 diabetes is being diagnosed at much earlier ages and much more frequently in Americans of all ages. Risk factors include a family history of diabetes, obesity, and a sedentary lifestyle. Type 2 diabetes typically has a much slower and less dramatic onset than type 1 diabetes and for this reason may persist for several years before people have symptoms that prompt them to seek medical care. Routine screening for diabetes is important and starts with a simple blood test. Although diabetes continues to be a challenging and life-altering condition, treatment has greatly improved.

In 1921, an orthopedist named Dr. Frederick Banting and his medical student assistant, Charles Best, began work on isolating insulin from the pancreas by studying dogs in the lab of J.J.R. Macleod in Toronto, Canada. In 1922, a 14-year-old boy who was dying from type 1 diabetes at the Toronto General Hospital was given the first injection of insulin harvested from a cow's pancreas. The patient suffered a severe allergic reaction, and further injections were postponed. The research team worked diligently to better purify the insulin extract and a second dose was injected. With this injection the sugar in the patient's urine disappeared, and the patient recovered with no obvious side effects. At a time when many people died from complications of type 1 diabetes, this extraordinary result must have seemed truly miraculous, particularly to all those affected by this disease. Banting and Macleod received the 1923 Nobel Prize in Physiology/Medicine and shared the award and recognition with their assistants, Charles Best and Bertram Collip. They made the patent readily available—without charge—and did not attempt to control the commercial production of insulin. In today's environment of pharmacologic patents worth hundreds of millions of dollars, such a scenario would be difficult to imagine.

The molecular structure of insulin was first determined by Frederick Sanger, who won the 1958 Nobel Prize in Chemistry for his work. Insulin was the first protein to have its sequence determined. The first genetically engineered "human" insulin was synthesized in a laboratory in 1977 by Genentech using the bacteria *Escherichia coli*. In 1982, biosynthetic human insulin became commercially available under the brand name Humulin. Biosynthetic insulin is now manufactured for widespread use via genetic engineering techniques using recombinant DNA technology.

Diabetes can be managed, and people with diabetes can have an excellent quality of life. A number of famous people have been affected by type 2 diabetes—Billie Jean King, Jackie Robinson, Dick Clark, Johnny Cash, Elvis Presley, and Larry King, to name a few. The Oscar-award winning actress Halle Berry, the 10-time Olympic medal swimmer Gary Hall Jr., and the musician Nick Jonas of the Jonas Brothers all developed type 1 diabetes as teenagers or young adults. Halle Berry is an active volunteer for the Juvenile Diabetes Association and Nick Jonas has developed the Change for the Children Foundation to raise money and awareness for diabetes.

DIABETES AND THE HAND: CONDITIONS AND TREATMENT

Diabetes can have an adverse effect on virtually every part of the body, including the hands. As a matter of fact, many conditions that manifest themselves in the hand are associated with diabetes. In addition, there are numerous hand conditions caused, exacerbated, or made more frequent by diabetes. Perhaps the best known is carpal tunnel syndrome. Although *carpal tunnel syndrome* (a compression of the median nerve where it passes through the wrist) often develops in people who do not have diabetes, the incidence among those with diabetes is significantly higher. (Carpal tunnel syndrome and its treatment are covered in chapter 9 of this book.)

Stenosing Tenosynovitis or Tendovaginitis ("Trigger Finger")

Stenosing tenosynovitis or tendovaginitis ("trigger finger") is when a person's finger is stuck, usually in a bent or flexed position, and it is quite difficult to straighten. It often appears after a person makes a fist, and one of the fingers remains bent when the fist is opened. The person has to work hard to straighten the finger, or must use the other hand to straighten it out. As the individual works to unbend the finger, it will usually release and suddenly straighten—that is, until a fist is made and it's stuck again. What is happening here? The tendon that bends the finger is getting stuck in its "pulley." With diabetes, the tendon and the pulley are more likely to swell, making it a tight fit for the tendon to move through the pulley. Picture a knot in your fishing line that gets caught in one of the eyes of the fishing pole and you have a good analogy.

Persons with diabetes are about 10 times more likely to experience a trigger digit than the rest of the population. Also, they more often have multiple trigger digits, meaning they may have several fingers that are triggering at any one time. Unfortunately, the typical nonsurgical treatments for trigger digit are less likely to be successful for people who have diabetes. And, as is the case for nearly all surgical procedures on people who have diabetes, there is a higher complication rate from trigger digit surgery for them, too.

That said, treatment options for trigger digit do include nonsurgical as well as surgical choices for those with diabetes. Nonsurgical measures can include activity modification, such as avoiding power-grip activities like gripping a hammer or cane too tightly. Splinting the digit straight can also be helpful and does prevent the finger from being flexed and getting stuck in that bent position. If splinting is used continuously for too long a period (more than about 4 to 6 weeks), however, the finger can become too stiff. If splinting is ineffective or the person prefers to bypass this option, the next nonsurgical choice is usually corticosteroid injections. The steroid, a very powerful anti-inflammatory, decreases the swelling of the tendon and its pulley, allowing the tendon to glide more freely. Unfortunately, this is one of the treatments for trigger digit that is much less effective in those with diabetes. While success rates of up to 85 percent or higher have been reported in the non-diabetic population, the success rates for steroid injections are often cited as 50 percent or below for persons with diabetes.

The surgical option for trigger finger is the same procedure for a person with diabetes as it is for anyone else. In surgery, an incision is made on the pulley where the tendon is caught, allowing the tendon to move freely through the area. The tendon is not trimmed; that could cause it to rupture. The tendon is what bends the finger, so if it were to be damaged the finger would not be able to bend.

There are two basic ways to do the surgery: open (with an incision) or percutaneous (under the skin). *Open surgery* is more common and starts with a small incision (about a half inch in length) on the palm of the hand. After the skin is opened, the pulley is identified and incised. *Percutaneous surgery* uses a needle or a thin scalpel to make a poke-hole in the skin and release the pulley in a "blind" fashion. The potential advantage here is that no skin incision is made, which may decrease infection risks as well as scarring and speed recovery time. The potential disadvantage, however, is that it is a "blind" procedure; the tendon and pulley are not directly seen, nor are the arteries and nerves that run past the tendon. This is concerning for many surgeons who fear that without direct visualization they may injure one or more of these structures. There may also not be a complete release of the pulley with this technique.

There are some minimally invasive options that use a fiber optic camera to make the process less "blind." Many hand surgeons prefer the open technique, however, because the potential risks of inadvertent harm with the minimally invasive percutaneous technique are too great.

Dupuytren Contracture

Dupuytren contracture (discussed in depth in chapter 10) is another disease in which the digits are held in a flexed position. But with Dupuytren contracture the digits cannot be pulled straight despite one's best efforts. The tissue in the hand and fingers that is usually soft and supple becomes hard and contracted, much like a thick scar. As tissue hardens and contracts on the palm side of the hand and digits, it draws them down into a flexed or bent position. Eventually, the fingers can be stuck in such a bent position that simple things like grabbing a cup or placing one's hands flat on a table are impossible. Despite its appearance, Dupuytren contracture is usually a painless condition (see figure 10.2). People of Northern European descent have the highest incidence of Dupuytren disease in the world.

People with diabetes, of any nationality, are more likely to develop Dupuytren contracture but the disorder is typically somewhat different for them. For example, Dupuytren contracture is usually present in the ring and small fingers of people who do not have diabetes, while those with diabetes are more likely to have it in the middle and ring fingers. Although we don't know why, Dupuytren disease tends to be less severe in persons with diabetes.

Treatment options for Dupuytren contracture are the same whether or not you have diabetes. Observation is the first step if the contracture is not painful or limiting hand function. Splints may be minimally helpful in limiting progression of contracture. If the disease is limiting function, more invasive treatment options can be considered. One quick way to determine if the disease is progressing significantly is to place your hand palm down on a table; if it can't be flattened, further medical attention should be sought. Surgery can involve complete opening of the palm and/or fingers and removing the scar tissue, or a more limited percutaneous approach. The decision to choose a more extensive or a limited approach is made based on a discussion with your surgeon.

Injections of enzymes that can dissolve the Dupuytren-affected tissue have been studied and are commercially available as the newest treatment option for Dupuytren disease. The medicine is injected into the Dupuytren-affected tissue on the first day, and the following day the finger is numbed and straightened as much as possible. Current studies show that this treatment is safer and has a faster recovery time than surgery in general but results in an earlier return of the disease on average, compared to surgery. It is best to get information on these different Dupuytren treatment options and discuss the pros and cons of each of them with your healthcare provider before selecting the method that is most appropriate for you.

Tendonitis/Tendonopathies ("Tennis Elbow" and Other Related Conditions)

People who have diabetes are more prone to develop *tendonitis*, which is inflammation of a tendon. One example of this condition is *de Quervain stenosing tenosynovitis*. Similar in concept to trigger finger, the location is different. De Quervain tenosynovitis occurs on the thumb side of the wrist, and pain is present when the thumb is pulled across the palm. In the past it was called *new mother's wrist*, and it may well be due to repeatedly picking up a newborn baby, but anyone can get de Quervain syndrome, from frequently lifting any heavy object in the way a baby is lifted. Traditional treatment options are similar to those for trigger finger: splint, anti-inflammatory medications, injection, or surgery. The splint must include the wrist and extend onto and around the thumb. It should surround the thumb, leaving only the last joint at the end of the thumb free to move. A regular wrist splint, one that does not include the thumb, will often make the symptoms worse because the splint stops right at the point of the problem, putting more pressure on the area.

Other examples of tendonitis/tendonopathies in diabetes include lateral *epicondylitis/epicondylopathy* ("tennis elbow") and *medial epicondylitis/epicondylopathy* ("golfer's elbow"). Surgical treatment, which involves releasing or removing the diseased tissue, is only rarely necessary for these two conditions.

Nerve Compression Syndromes (Other Than Carpal Tunnel Syndrome)

People with diabetes are more likely to develop nerve problems. This is why many of them develop carpal tunnel syndrome, as discussed earlier in this chapter. Other nerves in the arm and hand can also develop problems, and are more likely to do so if a person has diabetes. One of the more common nerve syndromes is cubital tunnel syndrome.

Cubital tunnel syndrome is a disease of the ulnar nerve at the elbow, commonly referred to as the "funny bone nerve." This nerve runs on the inside part of the elbow. When you strike your "funny bone," it is the ulnar nerve that has been hit and causes the tingling or burning sensation in the ring and small fingers. There is debate as to whether cubital tunnel syndrome is caused by the ulnar nerve being stretched or compressed or a combination of both. When you bend your elbow, pressure and traction on the ulnar nerve increase. It is thought that, over time, the ulnar nerve can become damaged through this repeated motion. There can be other reasons for increased pressure on the nerve, such as direct trauma, scarring, or deformity. Eventually, the tingling sensations in the ring and small fingers can become more severe and persistent, and even permanent if not addressed. Because the ulnar nerve also makes most of the muscles in the hand work, the grip and pinch strength of the hand can progressively deteriorate if the nerve is continually damaged.

Treatment options for cubital tunnel syndrome include activity modifications and splints to avoid direct trauma to the nerve and elbow flexion. Steroid injections are not usually used for cubital tunnel syndrome. If nonsurgical treatment doesn't work, or if the decreased sensation and hand weakness are severe, a doctor may recommend a surgical procedure to correct the problem. There are multiple surgical options and all of them work to take the pressure off the ulnar nerve at the elbow.

Infections

Well known to people with diabetes and those who care for them is their increased incidence of infections of all kinds. Not only are infections more common for people with diabetes, they also tend to be more severe and more difficult to treat. Infections of the hand are no different in this regard and need aggressive treatment; unfortunately, sometimes amputation is necessary when the infection will not heal. People who have diabetes are prone to a number of hand infections.

Felon. A *felon* is an infection of the pulp of the digit. Felons can start as a result of fingerstick sugar checks, which is why it is so important to clean the fingertip with alcohol and to use clean equipment when doing a fingerstick. A felon can be very painful and is typically swollen, red, and very tender to touch. The infection nearly always requires surgical drainage followed by wound care and antibiotics.

Paronychia. *Paronychia* refers to an infection of the skin that surrounds the fingernail. Typically the edges around the nail are swollen and red and may have pus drainage. If the infection is caught early, a regimen of warm water soaks and antibiotics can be effective. If left untreated or caught late, partial removal of the nail (at least) and surgical drainage are required. Even if the nail must be partially or completely removed, it will grow back unless the nail's growth cells have been severely damaged.

Infectious flexor tenosynovitis. *Infectious flexor tenosynovitis* is an infection of the tendons that bend the fingers. These tendons run through a tight tunnel. When an infection gets in, it is caught in a relatively enclosed space. The limited blood supply to this space means antibiotics are not very effective in getting to the infected area. Fingersticks or other wounds—especially puncture wounds such as animal bites—are often the initial cause of the infection. The finger will be swollen, very tender, and held in a bent position, and trying to straighten it will be very painful. If the infection continues untreated, permanent stiffness and tissue damage can occur. But if caught early, typically within 24 to 48 hours of onset and while the infection is relatively mild, a splint, elevation, intravenous antibiotics, and close observation in the hospital may be effective. It is not unusual for these infections to be treated in the operating room with a surgical "clean out" of the infected area. Once the infection is cleared, the focus becomes working out the stiffness and swelling the infection caused in the digit. This typically involves a relatively intense hand therapy program.

Fungal infections. People with diabetes are particularly prone to fungal infections. When these infections occur on or around the fingernails, they are termed *onychomycosis*. These infections can be difficult to eradicate and cause significant damage to the fingernails, which will become permanent if not treated early and effectively. Treatment medications may need to be continued for several weeks or even months, depending on the severity of the infection. Topical medications can be tried first if the infection is not too severe at the time of diagnosis. Medications taken by mouth can be more effective for more significant infections but can also be much more toxic. Liver function in particular needs to be checked before and during the treatment course if oral medications are used. Surgical treatment is usually reserved for more advanced and difficult cases. All or part of the nail is removed so that the organism causing the infection can be identified, allowing the doctor to prescribe medications that will clear the infection.

Vascular Disease ("Clogging of the Arteries")

People with diabetes have an increased risk of developing significant vascular disease. Diabetes causes damage to the large and small arteries throughout the body. Just like the heart, the hand and fingers can also be affected by this process. People with vascular disease in the hand will typically have pain because of poor blood flow to the hand and fingers. It is as if their hands are having a "heart attack." Along with pain, they may have a sensation of cold or tingling in the fingers. If the process continues or worsens they can develop wounds that do not heal and discoloration in their skin due to the decreased blood flow, usually starting at the tips of the fingers. The nails may also become discolored or develop dark streaks. Nonsurgical treatment options depend on the severity of the symptoms and the kind of physical changes that are occurring. Controlling glucose levels, stopping smoking, and avoiding cold environments are always good measures.

Your doctor may prescribe oral medications or injections around the fingers to try to increase blood flow and prevent clotting. When there is severe pain, non-healing ulcers, or impending tissue death, surgical intervention must be considered. The choice as to the type of procedure will depend on the timing of the process, the person's overall health status, and the condition of the arteries in the hand. Often, at this stage, an *arteriogram* is performed, a procedure similar to a cardiac catheterization in which a needle is placed into an artery in the thigh and guided up toward the heart. Dye is injected and an x-ray shows the dye running through the arteries into the arms, hands, and fingers, creating a "map" of the arteries and their vascular status (figures 8.1 and 8.2). Surgical options are often determined by an arteriogram map.

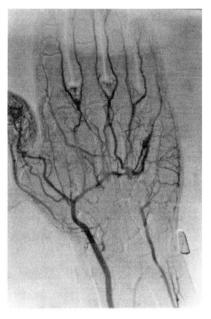

Stiff Hand

Persons with diabetes have a tendency to develop a stiff hand. This condition is often termed *limited joint mobility syndrome*, or *Rosenbloom syndrome*, and it is thought that only people who have diabetes develop it. When people with this syndrome try to put their hands together in a prayer-type position, a space can be seen between the two hands because they cannot be flattened

Figure 8.1. Angiogram showing blockage in ulnar artery. COURTESY THE CURTIS NATIONAL HAND CENTER

against each other. (This limitation is also seen with Dupuytren contracture; the difference is that usually not all digits are involved in Dupuytren contracture, and there are thick cords in the palm of the hand that are not present in limited joint mobility syndrome.)

Rosenbloom syndrome is distinct from the other possible causes of decreased range of motion of the hands in diabetes such as trigger digit and Dupuytren contracture. Those who develop Rosenbloom syndrome may also have stiff shoulders (a condition called *frozen shoulder* or the more technical term *adhesive capsulitis*). An increased incidence and severity of stiff hand syndrome has been correlated with older age,

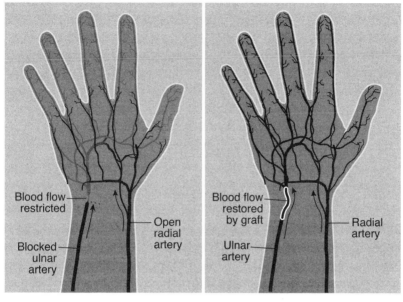

**Blood supply of left hand
with damaged ulnar artery**

**Blood supply of left hand
with bypassed ulnar artery**

Figure 8.2. Blood supply of left hand before and after surgical restoration of blood flow via grafting. ILLUSTRATION BY JACQUELINE SCHAFFER

male gender, longer duration of diabetes, and a poorer degree of glucose control. Treatments for this condition are largely nonsurgical and include control of any swelling, splinting as needed, and perhaps some medication alterations that should be discussed with an endocrinologist or primary care physician. Surgical treatment is only considered if there are significant limitations to the person's daily activities. In such cases, surgical release of tendons or joints may help.

Skin Changes

People with diabetes can have skin changes in the hands. Most of these are benign, painless conditions but they may be cosmetically troubling. The most common of these are *vitiligo* (loss or lack of pigmentation of the skin), *acanthosis nigricans* (hyperpigmentation of the skin), *bullosis diabeticorum* (skin blistering), and *necrobiosis lipoidica diabeticorum* (a rash that may itch or hurt and that is potentially the most severe condition, as painful ulcerations and infections may develop). An endocrinologist or primary care physician should be able to recognize the more common conditions, with referral to a dermatologist being needed only for more difficult or unusual situations.

◆

Individuals with diabetes should be seen by an endocrinologist, if at all possible, because these physicians have special expertise in the treatment of diabetes. If the need arises, an endocrinologist will likely also be able to refer you to a hand surgeon. In addition to the care of a medical expert, your own management of your diabetes is key to your health. You will find that nearly every hospital offers a variety of diabetes education, management, and support programs, most of which are covered by health insurance policies. Make note of what you have learned in this chapter and take advantage of these programs. Your efforts will greatly determine your quality of life and protect those essential tools of living: your hands.

CHAPTER 9

SENSE AND SENSIBILITY

◆

*Seeing the World with Braille and Understanding
Nerve Impairment Syndromes*

Ryan M. Zimmerman, M.D., and Neal B. Zimmerman, M.D.

In many ways, Mrs. Johnson was typical of patients who come to our hand clinic. She was in her mid-forties and dressed casually, in jeans and sweater. She brought along her support system, her sister and her daughter, who were quietly seated in a corner of the exam room. But that was where typical ended.

"Doctor, you've got to help me," Mrs. Johnson pleaded, clasping her hands together. "I'm going blind."

Why, you might be wondering, *was she consulting a hand surgeon?*

Mrs. Johnson (not her real name) had lost the last remnants of her sight in both eyes decades earlier. She was in our hand clinic not because of anything to do with her eyes but because of numbness and tingling in her fingertips. As her quivering voice made clear, the hand has unique importance for the person who has seriously impaired vision.

When a person's vision falters, the human hand takes on many tasks that were once performed by the eyes. When that person's hands' ability to move or to sense the outside world also wavers, she is left doubly disabled because the most important alternative means of perception and communication has been lost.

We don't know exactly how many Americans suffer from both vision loss and upper extremity sensory problems. We do know that in 2006, the National Health Interview Survey determined that 21.2 million Americans suffer from significant vision loss, unable to see well enough to perform daily tasks despite corrective glasses or contacts. Of this group, approximately 6.2 million were senior citizens. Although these figures are daunting, the numbers are likely to increase in the near future. Right behind the more than 6 million currently vision-impaired senior citizens are 9 million "baby boomers" with some degree of vision loss, which means that the number of older Americans with poor vision will increase substantially in the coming decades. And blindness is a problem spanning all generations: there are nearly 58,000 legally blind children in America today.

There are many reasons for vision loss: age-related changes (*macular degeneration*), pressure inside the eye (*glaucoma*), trauma, congenital conditions, inherited disease, infection, and strokes. And, there are just as many medical conditions that cause sensory difficulties in the hands, affecting the nerves that relay information through our palms and fingers back to the brain about the objects we encounter or the hand's position in space. While several such problems are illustrated in this chapter, one condition must be mentioned at the outset. Despite its ancient roots, diabetes remains one of medicine's greatest challenges and is the main cause of simultaneous vision and sensory nerve dysfunction.

The American Diabetes Association defines *diabetes* simply as "a disease in which the body does not produce or properly use insulin." As described in chapter 8, *insulin* is a hormone produced by the pancreas that causes the body's cells to take up and use sugar molecules (glucose) from the blood. When the body makes too little insulin or doesn't respond to it correctly, glucose levels build up. And when blood sugar levels remain too high for a long time, tissues throughout the body are damaged via complex and varied mechanisms, including impaired oxygen delivery and inflammation.

Diabetes frequently affects the peripheral nerves that carry sensation from the hands to the spinal cord, which then transmits those impulses to several specific areas of the brain. In the United States, 23.6 million people suffer from diabetes and 57 million have what is referred to as "pre-diabetes," which means they show signs of the disease without fitting all the diagnostic criteria. Unfortunately, nearly one-quarter of people with diabetes don't know they have it, so their bodies are sustaining damage they don't even know is occurring.

While the complications of diabetes include heart disease, stroke, and kidney disease, it is also the leading cause of new cases of blindness in adults aged 20 to 74 years, with *diabetic retinopathy*, one form of diabetic eye disease, causing 12,000 to 24,000 new cases of blindness annually, according to the U.S. Centers for Disease Control. Furthermore, 60 to 70 percent of individuals with diabetes have some form of neurological impairment, such as poor sensation in the hands or carpal tunnel syndrome. These numbers mean there are at least 14.2 million Americans with nervous system dysfunction and at least 12,000 new cases of blindness each year due to diabetes. Understanding the unique role of the hands for vision-impaired individuals is more than just an intellectual exercise. Examining what the hand is called on to do when vision fails helps us understand how the hands become the "eyes" for people who are blind. Knowing which sensory functions of the hands must be restored for a blind individual to use his hands to "see" again prepares physicians to treat those individuals.

When most of us think about the new tasks the hands take on when a person cannot see, reading comes to mind first. Learning to read and write Braille is an incredible task charged to the hands but one that allows blind persons the opportunity to exist with a greater degree of independence. To understand why the Braille alphabet works is to understand the way the hand works. The story of Braille is a marvel of human ingenuity and determination—starring the sensitivity of our fingertips.

THE BIRTH OF BRAILLE

A common misconception is that Braille was the first attempt to develop a way for blind people to read. The fact is numerous other approaches had been tried first, from magnifying individual letters when a little visual ability remained (either through the use of magnifying glasses for regular books or by printing books with extra large type) to raised versions of the unchanged printed alphabet characters. But these approaches shared the same fundamental flaw common to many early schemes: they were adaptations of a vision-based system, instead of being built on the unique characteristics of the hand. The role of the hand in blindness is not just to assume the tasks of the eye as closely as it can but to modify the way those tasks are accomplished to fit its nuances and special abilities. By appreciating this relationship, the beauty and elegance of how the human hand has adopted and shaped the world of the blind is all the more impressive.

The history of Braille, like the history of most things, is about more than just the superficial facts. The real story of the Braille alphabet is its inventor, Louis Braille, a brilliant young boy whose intellect, creativity, and desire to learn have improved the world for millions of blind people.

Louis Braille was born in 1810, with normal vision and a sharp mind, the son of a saddle-maker in the French village of Coupvray, 30-some miles east of Paris. At the age of 3, Louis was playing in his father's workshop when he accidentally struck himself in the eye with one of the tools. He became blind in the injured eye and, worse, he subsequently lost vision in the other eye as well through what was likely *sympathetic ophthalmia*, an incompletely understood process in which the body attacks a normal, healthy eye after injury to its partner.

Even without sight, Louis continued to hunger for knowledge; at the age of 10 he earned a scholarship to the Parisian National Institute for the Blind. There, vision-impaired children were taught trade skills as well as how to read using a system of raised but otherwise unaltered letters. While such a technique could technically allow blind people to read, it required tracing the shape of each letter with the fingertips. Because of the size of each letter and the weight of the books (sometimes more than 100 pounds), reading was slow and Louis remained frustrated. Then, in 1821, a French Army captain by the name of Charles Barbier visited the school and provided Louis with the inspiration he needed.

During his visit, Captain Barbier taught the children a military code called Night Writing, initially designed to help sighted soldiers secretly share information on the battlefield. This system was unique; instead of relying on three-dimensional, raised reproductions of letters and numbers, the alphanumeric characters were encoded using a grid system.

The Night Writing grid was a six-by-two dot matrix, where the arrangement of raised dots corresponded to a particular letter or number. While this method was a significant improvement, it was still inadequate. It was only through an understanding of how the hands actually read that Louis Braille, then just 11 years old, was able to make subtle but crucial adjustments to the Night Writing code that yielded the Braille alphabet.

Although blind people could more easily discern Night Writing dots than they could raised letters, both approaches shared a fundamental flaw: neither could convey all of its information to a reader's fingertip with a single impression. Just as an embossed letter required the reader's fingertip to travel across its curves and angles, so too the Night Writing code required multiple impressions on the fingertip to traverse its six rows. Louis Braille understood this limitation and changed the Night Writing code to a three-row by two-column cell of dots that we now know as the Braille alphabet. A seemingly minor change, Braille's simplicity is equaled only by its brilliance. It represented a completely new understanding of how the hand works when we ask it to read.

Up to this point, the emphasis had been on training the finger to read exactly like the eye, which was a natural but flawed approach. Unlike the eye, the fingertip is a highly precise tool that is most efficient when stationary. Moving the hand around while feeling across multiple rows of dots or along the ridges of an embossed letter requires the brain to put together all of the various pieces of sensory information to reconstruct the entire perceived object—a highly complex task that takes time and precious mental energy away from focusing on the meaning of what is written. The fingertip, however, is highly adept at discerning between two closely located points (figure 9.1). By exploiting these unique characteristics of the human hand, and respecting its limitations, Louis Braille was able to make a condensed, quickly read alphabet that still works today (figure 9.2).

A total of 63 combinations can be made from the 6-dot matrix, far more permutations than the number of letters in European alphabets. Louis used an easy-to-learn system to decide which patterns would correspond to letters. The first 10 letters of the alphabet (*A–J*) are all formed using only the top 2 rows of dots. Beginning with the letter *K*, the bottom row of dots comes into play. For the next 10 letters, the same

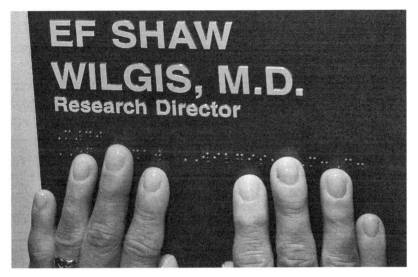

Figure 9.1. Braille being read with two hands. COURTESY NORMAN H. DUBIN, PH.D.

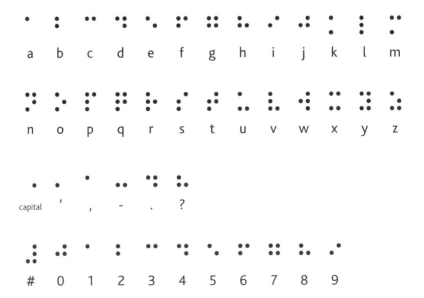

Figure 9.2. The Braille alphabet and numbers. ADAPTED FROM THE AMERICAN FOUNDATION FOR THE BLIND (HTTP://BRAILLEBUG.AFB.ORG) USING THE BRAILLE FONT KAEDING BRAILLE.

cycle is repeated on the top 2 rows, while the bottom left dot is added. Then, again, the same cycle is repeated on the top with the bottom right dot added. The letter *w* is an exception because the French alphabet didn't include this letter until years after Louis invented his alphabet.

Why did Louis Braille, and everyone who came before him, choose the hands as the medium for reading the alphabet? The answer illustrates both our reliance on our hands and our tendency to take them for granted: touch is quick, reproducible, and fairly unobjectionable in a way that other sensory modalities are not. Exploring why our hands get charged with so many, and such varied, tasks tells us a great deal about the human hand, as well as its vulnerabilities and its unique role in the lives of the blind.

THE AMAZING 2-MILLIMETER 2-POINT DISCRIMINATION

We rely on our hands because of several important physiologic factors: hands are mobile and dexterous, and have highly developed sensory capabilities. The hands and arms have no weight-bearing role during walking (unlike in many other animals), so they are free to assume other responsibilities and be used in skills other than mobility. But one of the most interesting characteristics about the hands is the one that is absolutely required to read Braille and often missing for people with nerve injury: *2 millimeter 2-point discrimination*. What this means is that the hands, and especially the fingertips, can differentiate between two stimuli that are only 2 millimeters apart! If you think that 2 millimeters is a small distance, take a ruler and measure the distance between the dots on Braille letters—you may be surprised by just how small the distance is.

While 2-point discrimination may seem at first to be an awkward way to measure sensibility, it is actually quite intuitive since the basic question being asked of any group of sensory nerves is whether something is there. *Is there a hot stove touching my finger or is there not?* Once that question has been answered, 2-point discrimination indicates how precisely the location of that stimulus is known to be present or absent. For example, telling someone your house number is more precise than giving her only the street name; 2-point discrimination gives the finger-tip an objective way to measure sensory perception. Its deterioration can indicate a sensory nerve injury.

If you have any doubt that the sense of touch on your fingertips is more precise than elsewhere on your body, try this. Take a household item with two points located a small distance from one another (such as a fine-tooth comb). With your eyes closed, press the points lightly onto your fingertip (a common mistake among new Braille readers is press-ing too hard). Count the number of discrete points you feel while some-one else watches how many points are making contact. Then, move to your lip, another very sensitive spot, and repeat. Now, repeat this same test on your lower back and on the back of your thigh. How accurate were you? Was there any difference? Most people note excellent ac-curacy using their fingertips and lips, but significantly less along their lumbar spine or posterior thigh, and this is because of the difference in 2-point discrimination between these sites. The physiological factors at work are the different density of sensory nerve fibers in these regions of your body, as well as the amount of brain tissue dedicated to sensory perception for each of these areas.

Relative to their actual size, the hands and face are disproportion-ately represented in the brain, which corresponds to their unique sensory abilities (and to their success in the test you just performed). Multiple experiments have shown the ability of brain tissue, such as that within the visual cortex at the back of the brain (usually responsible for sight), to be reprogrammed in blind people to functions associated with touch and sign language. Although these facts are fascinating and help to explain how and why sighted and blind people alike have come to rely on the hand, they also set the stage for understanding the devastating nature of sensory nerve problems in the hands.

PINCHED NERVES

The most common cause of nerve dysfunction is external compression of peripheral nerves, rather than neuropathy due to diabetes. Peripheral nerves are very much like television or Internet cables: a signal is created at one end and carried along its length to a receiver that turns the signal into meaningful content. Like television and Internet cables, peripheral nerves are susceptible to physical damage (such as when a digging crew cuts into a cable line) or chemical damage (such as when copper wires rust). A typical peripheral nerve like the *median nerve* (which primarily connects to the thumb, index finger, and middle finger) is composed of tens of thousands of microscopic fibers. The metabolic portion of a sensory nerve, its *cell body*, is located in the spinal cord, quite a distance from the area it is responsible for sensing.

A single nerve can be several feet long, running from the neck to the fingertip. The long, extended portion of the nerve is called the *axon*, and it houses an insulated electrical system (similar to that used in modern electrical wires) designed to deliver minute electrical impulses to the spinal cord and from there up into the brain. Normal joint movements or body positions will stretch or pinch nerves to a mild degree. Consider where the ulnar nerve passes behind the large bone on the inside of your elbow; arm movements pinch and stretch the nerve as it runs across the elbow.

Such physical influences are mostly unperceivable. In certain situations, however, physical compression or tension on a nerve is quite obvious. One example is when your hand "falls asleep" or you "hit your funny bone." In the former the median nerve has been compressed, while in the latter the ulnar nerve has been physically struck.

Although both diabetic neuropathies and compressive neuropathies (*neuropathy* is a broad term that refers to any nerve abnormality) can cause numbness and tingling, the root causes are quite different. In *diabetic neuropathy*, the surrounding structures are fine and interact with the nerve without difficultly. The problem lies within the nerve's metabolism. In *compressive neuropathy* the nerve itself is intrinsically working well, but because it is pathologically pinched or stretched, it will eventually begin to function poorly. Pinching or stretching of the nerve slowly and gradually degrades its ability to convey impulses to the spinal cord and brain at the correct speed and with the correct strength.

Carpal tunnel syndrome is by far the most common compressive neuropathy in the arms and hands. It is so prevalent that the diagnosis is sometimes made based only a patient's history and physical examination, without any neurologic testing. The term *carpal tunnel syndrome* refers to a specific process in which the median nerve (the one that provides sensation to the thumb, index finger, and middle finger) is compressed as it passes through a small bony and fibrous channel at the base of the wrist (figure 9.3). This channel is called the *carpal tunnel* because the bones that form much of its boundaries are collectively referred to as the carpal bones. Carpal tunnel syndrome is typified by numbness and tingling in the thumb, index finger, and middle finger, causing discomfort that frequently awakens a person from sleep. This problem is most common in women, and at approximately the time of menopause.

Doctors used to think (as much of the lay public still does) that the most common reason for compressive neuropathy such as carpal tunnel was repetitive activity, such as typing. Researchers, however, have found little evidence to support this theory. Arguably, the majority of hand surgeons believe the predominant reasons for compressive neuropathy are anatomic variations, aging, and fluid shifts due to menopause. Only a small portion of carpal tunnel syndrome cases, if any, are attributable to repetitive activity or the use of keyboards.

Carpal tunnel syndrome is the most common cause of sensation loss in the hand. In addition to providing sensation to the thumb, index finger, and middle finger, the median nerve also controls the small muscles around the base of the thumb. Therefore, in severe cases of carpal tunnel syndrome, the person experiences difficulty positioning the thumb and performing precise pinching activities. As sensation in the hand wanes, fine tasks such as threading a needle or buttoning clothing become increasingly difficult. If the condition goes on for too long, the person will experience more clumsiness as even gross motor skills—holding a cup, bathing, or cooking—slowly deteriorate.

Carpal tunnel syndrome is usually diagnosed by a combination of a clinical examination and electrodiagnostic testing that graphs the transmission of impulses along the nerve. The initial treatment for carpal tunnel syndrome is usually the use of a splint at night, as well as oral medications or injections to help restore the local anatomy to normal. If carpal tunnel syndrome is severe or fails to resolve with nonsurgical means, surgery is frequently recommended.

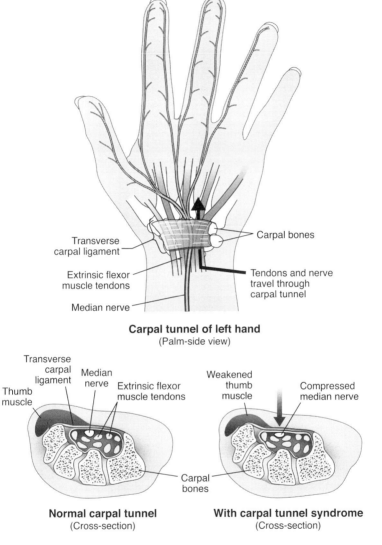

Transverse
carpal ligament

Extrinsic flexor
muscle tendons

Median nerve

Carpal bones

Tendons and nerve
travel through
carpal tunnel

Carpal tunnel of left hand
(Palm-side view)

Transverse
carpal
ligament

Thumb
muscle

Median
nerve

Extrinsic flexor
muscle tendons

Weakened
thumb
muscle

Compressed
median nerve

Carpal
bones

Normal carpal tunnel
(Cross-section)

With carpal tunnel syndrome
(Cross-section)

Figure 9.3. Carpal tunnel of the hand. ILLUSTRATION BY JACQUELINE SCHAFFER

The aim of carpal tunnel surgery is to increase the size of the carpal tunnel, thus relieving pressure on the median nerve and providing it with an opportunity to heal. After surgery, people often note that sensation in their hands returns rapidly. In severe or longstanding cases of carpal tunnel syndrome, damage to the nerve and the muscles it controls may be permanent. Sensory return and muscle regeneration may be only partial, and the recovery quite prolonged.

Within the past decade, there have been impressive advances in the surgical treatment of carpal tunnel syndrome. Previously, carpel tunnel surgery entailed a large incision in the center of the palm. This approach was effective in relieving pressure on the median nerve but, due to the size of the incision, recovery time was substantial. With recent advances, carpal tunnel surgery can now be performed using an incision less than an inch long. The median nerve is still adequately decompressed, and post-procedure hand tenderness is minimal.

A question that comes up time and again is whether a person needs to stop a particular activity to make the carpal tunnel syndrome resolve, even following surgery. There is little, if any, evidence to support this concern. The most common cause of recurrent or persistent carpal tunnel syndrome is an inaccurate initial diagnosis. Such confusion often arises because of the symptom overlap in the hands due to compression of several different nerves in various locations, ranging from the wrist to the elbow to the spine. Furthermore, the popularity and success of carpal tunnel surgery causes some patients to push for the procedure as a perceived cure, even when their symptoms are inconsistent with a diagnosis of carpal tunnel syndrome.

Carpal tunnel syndrome is the most common compression neuropathy in the upper extremity; compression of the ulnar nerve at the elbow is the runner-up. The *ulnar nerve* runs just behind the bone on the inside of the elbow (the medial humeral epicondyle) and down to the small and ring fingers. In addition to the sensation it provides to the small and ring fingers, the ulnar nerve also controls the majority of the small muscles in the hand. The symptoms of ulnar neuropathy at the elbow are distinct from those of carpal tunnel. People with compression of the ulnar nerve at the elbow frequently complain of numbness and tingling in the small and ring fingers and also have difficulty spreading their fingers apart and pulling them together or with forceful pinching with the thumb.

Ulnar neuropathy at the elbow usually causes numbness in the small and ring fingers when the elbow is resting on a table or the armrest of a car. The numbness radiates from the inside part of the elbow down to the small and ring fingers.

Usually, the ulnar nerve is loosely bound in a bony groove along the inside of the elbow. With elbow flexion, the nerve moves forward and is both stretched across and pressed against the back of the *medial epicondyle*, the bony structure at the elbow behind which the nerve runs. With time, this stretching and pressing can cause changes in the nerve, resulting in altered function. In some individuals, however, the nerve is more mobile, and actually slips over the medial epicondyle onto the wrong side during elbow flexion, causing further trauma.

Nonsurgical treatment of ulnar neuropathy at the elbow begins with a splint to keep the elbow semi-extended and allow the nerve to recover from being stretched and compressed against the medial epicondyle. If nonsurgical treatment fails, there are a variety of surgical procedures that cure the problem by moving the ulnar nerve to the front of the elbow to prevent it from being further damaged.

REFERRED PAIN

Although peripheral nerve disease that affects the hand can originate in the wrist or elbow, it is important to note that the nerves controlling the upper extremities originate in the brain and cervical spinal cord. Symptoms in the hand can be caused by disease at these more distant locations. A concept in medicine that is especially relevant in a field such as hand surgery is that of *referred pain*, which is when a problem at one place (such as the cervical spine) manifests as pain elsewhere (such as the hand).

The nerve roots that eventually course down to the hand can be compressed as they exit the spinal cord through small openings between the vertebrae that form the spinal column. These small openings between vertebrae, called *neural foramina*, can become tightened, a process referred to as *stenosis*, through several mechanisms. There are six small joints at almost every spinal level, and these joints can become arthritic, just like any other joint in the body. The most common type of arthritis—*osteoarthritis*—develops when the cartilage, which provides cushioning and the low-friction gliding surface of the joint, wears out. In an attempt to increase the gliding surface and distribute the stress from loss of the cartilage cushion, bony material is added at the edges of a joint, right where the neural foraminae are located. This extra bone is often referred to as *bone spurs*, or *osteophytes*. The size of the neural foramina can be compromised as these osteophytes invade the space typically reserved for the foraminae, thus compressing the nerve roots as they exit the spinal cord.

But there are still more places where the nerves are subject to injury on their trip from the brain to the fingertip. The nerve roots go through a branching and melding process on their way down to the hand; the fibers that comprise the nerves that run through the wrist or elbow consist of nerve fibers emanating from several different levels in the spine. Therefore, the same nerves that are involved with carpal tunnel syndrome or ulnar neuropathy can exit the cervical spine successfully but get compressed because of disease in the shoulder or chest (such as trauma from a skiing accident or a tumor at the top of the lung) that violates the nerve fibers as they come together to form the final nerves in an anatomical structure referred to as the *brachial plexus*.

Finally, disease at one site does not prevent problems from developing elsewhere. Cervical spinal nerve root compression can occur alone or can coexist with compression of either the median or ulnar nerve. Frequently, identifying the location of nerve impingement requires electrodiagnostic studies, MRI (magnetic resonance imaging) scans, and a careful physical examination.

Treatment of cervical spine disease is often nonsurgical, relying on a combination of physical therapy and medication. The symptoms of cervical spine disease differ from those of carpal tunnel syndrome and ulnar neuropathy. Neck pain is commonly associated with numbness in the hand; a careful physical examination can sometimes ferret out that only part of the median nerve is involved. Since multiple nerves exit from the spine to form the median nerve, only some of them may have spinal disease. Surgical treatment is sometimes required to remove the bone spurs pressing on the nerve roots, and may include fusing together several spinal segments to provide more room for the nerve roots as they exit the vertebral column.

CONDITIONS OF THE BRAIN

While the spine may seem to be located too far from the hand to cause such localized symptoms, there are even higher sites of disease that must be considered when a person has hand problems. *Multiple sclerosis* is a condition that differs from the other neuropathies discussed thus far for two reasons. First, its origin is central, arising directly from the brain. Second, all of the other processes discussed thus far share some element of physical compression (at the wrist, elbow, or spine), and there is no element of physical compression in multiple sclerosis. This disease causes scattered injuries to various brain regions, possibly through an autoimmune process where the body's immune system attacks its own brain tissue. These lesions disrupt the perception of the neural impulses carried from the hand (leading to numbness), as well as impulses carried from the brain distally (causing weakness or clumsiness). Multiple sclerosis often first manifests as decreased sensibility in the hands or dysfunction of the eyes. Anyone who has numbness in the hands needs to undergo a full neurologic examination to determine the location of the problem.

TRAUMA

If there seems to be an impressive array of ways in which nerves can be injured from within the human body, that there are even more ways to injure them from outside. The possibilities include knives, bullets, broken glass, animal bites, burns, automobiles, and literally thousands of other traumatic injuries.

Nerve trauma is akin to the division of a large fiber optic cable carrying tens of thousands of fibers. The body's initial reaction to a nerve laceration is to mobilize scavenger cells to remove the dead or damaged parts of the nerve, leaving the scaffolding (the myelin sheaths) intact. The scavenging and pruning back of the traumatized portion of the nerves is referred to as *Wallerian degeneration*. Following nerve laceration, the *proximal* (near) end of the nerve sprouts forth like the roots of a tree, attempting to reestablish a connection with the other end of the tubes where they previously resided. A complex interplay of chemicals is excreted from the far ends of the nerve to attract the growing nerve fibers to its distant targets, as well as from the near end of the interrupted nerve to stimulate growth. This process of nerve growth is slow. Its tortoise-like pace is responsible for the long healing times required for nerve injuries. Once the nerve fibers connect with their intended targets, many of the side branches are trimmed or pruned and the connections that are successfully reconnected are reinforced.

Surgical nerve repair in the extremities is more a realignment of the ends of the nerve to guide the sprouting axons to their targeted myelin sheaths than a mechanical process like sewing the nerve ends together. Surgeons are finding success, however, with a new type of biologic glue, called *fibrin glue*, and using it for direct nerve repair. Recent research has reported that nerve regeneration is more effective if there is a very small gap left between the tips of the nerve ends to allow them to sprout, reconnect, and prune their connections through the natural process. If the ends are forced too tightly together and not allowed to find their way naturally, the nerve fibers do not have an opportunity to branch and find their targets with the same degree of efficiency. Indeed, it seems that no matter how advanced technology gets, natural processes cannot necessarily be surpassed. Case in point: the most important factor in recovery of function following a nerve injury is a person's age. The most skilled surgeon cannot replace the ability of a younger nerve to seek its targets more vigorously than a more aged nerve.

Although nature may know best, modern medicine is doing an admirable job trying to keep up. There has been a great deal of research using dissolvable synthetic tubes to guide the ends of regenerating nerves toward each other. Another new avenue of research is the transfer of functional nerves from one part of the body to reconnect to targets when the original nerve is not available to do so. For example, surgeons have successfully rerouted nerves from under the ribs to provide motion to a paralyzed arm.

To truly understand the human hand, we must learn to see our hands for what they are: highly precise, integrated machines whose health and function extend from the brain to the fingertips. Although it is easy to take our hands for granted, just as we do our ability to breathe, when you take a moment to think about the importance of the human hand in the way we experience our world, you may experience a stunning realization.

Blind people show us that the human hand is almost always up to whatever task it is charged with. The tragic accident that blinded Louis Braille as a young boy led him to develop a language we read with our fingertips—a luminous testament to the fact that there is no limit to what the hand can do. The only thing we can know for sure is that the human hand will always find new ways to carry us forward, as individuals and as a society.

CHAPTER 10

THE RENOIR EFFECT

◆

Contractures and Spasticity

Christopher L. Forthman, M.D.

When the hand is healthy and fully functional, it can reflect a person's occupation, mental skills, and emotions. At a glance, you may be able to discern the farmer from the hair stylist from the professor from the chef from the yoga instructor—just by looking at the person's hands. Most of the time, that is.

Anyone meeting Auguste Renoir (the famous impressionist painter) for the first time later in the artist's life would never guess the man to be a fine arts painter. Rheumatoid arthritis caused severely deforming and crippling contracture of Renoir's hands, making them appear useless. With the help of an assistant, however, who would place a paint brush in the artist's closed, gnarled hand, Renoir created some of his most famous works during the last 25 years of his life—the period when the rheumatoid arthritis in his hands had progressed to its worst stage (figure 10.1).

When the hand suffers from the diseases of contracture or spasticity, its appearance and function cannot fully express the whole person. And when hand contractures or spasticity are severe, the condition can leave the person unable to work or even care for himself. The problems caused by contracture or spasticity lead to alterations in the hand's form as much as its function. Fortunately, today there are better treatments

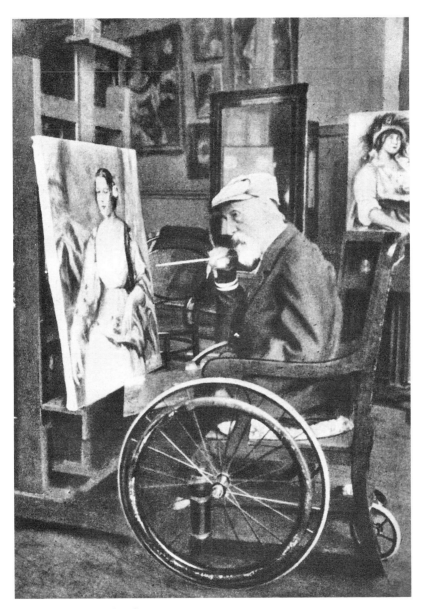

Figure 10.1. Auguste Renoir

than ever before that address these disorders. Some of the conditions that follow have been mentioned in earlier chapters; here they are explored in more detail.

DUPUYTREN DISEASE

Dupuytren contracture is a slowly progressive tissue contracture in the palm that results in a fixed, flexed position of the fingers, especially the ring and small fingers (figure 10.2). The condition bears the name *Dupuytren disease* after the French surgeon Baron Guillaume Dupuytren, who in 1832 developed a surgical procedure to correct it. The "papal benediction sign" (where the fourth and fifth fingers are contracted) may reveal the hand deformity of a pope who lived long ago.

Dupuytren disease affects men more often than women and usually does not begin to develop until middle age. A particularly severe form of the disease can have an earlier onset and is associated with contractures of the feet and penis as well.

The exact cause of Dupuytren disease is unknown. There is speculation that trauma, epilepsy, liver disease, smoking, and alcohol use may predispose a person to Dupuytren disease but no definitive relationship has ever been proven. What is happening biologically, however, is well understood: cells proliferate excessively and produce fibrous tissue that thickens and contracts the tissue under the skin of the palm and fingers. Nodules and dimples may appear, along with cords running from the palm into the fingers. As the contractures progress, the person is not able to fully open his hand.

We do know that Dupuytren disease has a genetic predisposition, sometimes running in families and generally occurring in persons of Scandinavian or Northern European descent. In fact, Dupuytren disease has the nickname "Viking" or "Celtic" disease, reflecting the prevalence of this problem in populations that once fell under the influence of Norsemen. Historical writing and artwork, however, suggests that Dupuytren disease was seen before the era of the Vikings.

Today, Dupuytren disease is rare, affecting only about 5 percent of the population. Yet the disease is familiar to many because it has been diagnosed in Ronald Reagan, Margaret Thatcher, and other well-known public figures. We also see Dupuytren contracture on the "big screen"— the British actor Bill Nighy, the pop star Bill Mack in *Love Actually*, and David McCallum (Dr. "Ducky" Mallard on *NCIS*) are just a few examples of Hollywood stars with Dupuytren disease.

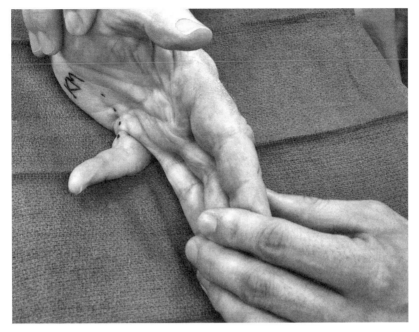

Figure 10.2. Dupuytren contracture. COURTESY KENNETH R. MEANS JR., M.D.

Fortunately, Dupuytren contractures do not usually cause pain. Most people affected have minimal contractures and are able to live with the disease untreated. Those with substantial contracture, however, often have difficulty opening the hand for grasping or placing the hand in a pocket or glove, playing a musical instrument, or participating in sports. Today, these functional limitations can be addressed by surgical procedures to release or remove the contracted tissues.

Treatment for Dupuytren Contracture

The first surgery for Dupuytren contracture was performed by Baron Guillaume Dupuytren in 1832 and involved a simple division (loosening) of the tight cords. Since then, surgeons have focused on segmental or complete removal of the diseased tissue. More recently, percutaneous mechanical or chemical methods to release the contracted bands have been developed. Currently, there is debate within the medical community about the best treatment for the disease. In general, nonsurgical or minimally invasive procedures offer a quicker recovery, while surgical excision of the contracted tissue may be more successful in reducing the risk of recurrence of the disease.

Needle aponeurotomy (NA) or *fasciotomy* is a minimally invasive technique directed at straightening bent fingers to make them functional again. The procedure is done under local anesthesia and uses a small needle to make a series of cuts in the contracted tissue under the skin. Immediate motion is possible because there are usually no open wounds. A splint is worn after the procedure (especially at night) for up to 3 months to help straighten the fingers. While the risk of recurrence with NA can be higher than with more invasive techniques, advocates of NA point out that the procedure is fairly painless, has a fast recovery, and can be repeated if necessary. Because this procedure is done "blindly," some surgeons avoid it due to the risk of inadvertent injury to other structures in the hand such as nerves, blood vessels, and tendons.

The diseased bands of tissue can also be released by "melting" a portion of the cord with an enzyme called *Clostridial collagenase*. The procedure is similar to needle aponeurotomy in that the restrictive bands are disrupted. But unlike with NA, with enzyme injection, the bands are dissolved slowly. Splinting is used to accelerate separation of the diseased tissue. Phase III clinical trials of Clostridial collagenase were recently completed in the United States and results published in the *New England Journal of Medicine* are encouraging. As with all procedures, the possibility of inadvertently dissolving an important structure such as a tendon remains a concern.

Excision (surgical removal) of the diseased tissue is known as *fasciectomy*. Both partial (segmental) excision and complete (radical) fasciectomy have been advocated. Sometimes the adherent skin overlying the nodules and cords is removed as well. In any of these approaches, the goal is to remove the disease and reduce the rate of recurrence. These wounds are slow to heal after surgery, and most patients need the help of a hand therapist to regain motion during the recovery period. Open surgery, like the minimally invasive techniques, may also result in injury to other structures in the hand—particularly nerves that become wrapped up in the cords of severe contractures. In particularly severe cases of Dupuytren contracture, skin grafts may be necessary.

POST-TRAUMATIC CONDITIONS

Ischemic Contracture

Trauma to the hand and arm can result in varying degrees of fixed contracture. A particularly severe post-traumatic condition was described by Dr. Richard von Volkmann in 1881, implicating loss of blood supply as a cause of flexor muscle death in the forearm. The term *Volkmann ischemic contracture* eventually came to identify a fixed flexion posture to the wrist and fingers following a fracture, excessively tight bandage, or arterial damage. Most cases in the early literature focused on contractures in children after bone breaks in the elbow and forearm.

The underlying cause of ischemic contracture is increased pressure in a muscle compartment, a phenomenon known as *compartment syndrome*. Today, compartment syndrome in the hand and forearm is usually associated with crush injuries or severe bone fractures. Such a high degree of trauma involves considerable force, as you might experience in a car crash. Earthquakes, like the 2010 disaster in Haiti, are notorious for causing devastating crush injuries with damage to both soft tissue and bone. Whatever the cause, the results are increased muscle pressures and decreased blood flow. Muscle tissue dies, contracts, and forms deep scars, keeping the hand and wrist from moving. Nerves may also stop functioning, leading to loss of feeling and additional muscle dysfunction. In the worst cases, the hand and wrist adopt a flexed, claw-like posture.

Treatment for ischemic contracture. The best treatment for Volkmann ischemic or compartment syndrome–related contracture begins with early recognition of the problem. Prompt diagnosis and treatment will prevent most cases from developing into permanent contracture. The affected person often complains of severe pain, exceeding the level of pain expected for the injury. Pain worsens with any attempt to move the fingers. In addition, the hand and arm appear swollen and feel tight. Pressures in the forearm and hand can be measured by a doctor to confirm the diagnosis.

Immediate treatment includes the removal of tight bandages and casts; on occasion, swollen muscular compartments require emergency surgery to release the pressure. If muscle death occurs, therapy and splinting to minimize contracture will be started. When severe contractures do develop, function can often be improved with surgery to release scar tissue, reroute healthy tendons from another part of the arm, and even transfer muscle from another part of the body to the forearm and hand.

There are many other traumas besides compartment syndrome that can result in contractures. In fact, most loss of hand function after trauma is a "normal" or "expected" consequence of the injury sustained. For example, knife injuries often cause lacerations of nerves and tendons. These structures can be repaired surgically but rarely regain full function. Tendons fail to glide smoothly and become trapped in beds of scar tissue while nerves short-circuit and fail to transmit adequate electrical signals. Similarly, direct damage to joints—from any injury or disease—can lead to loss of motion. Physical and occupational therapists can help the injured person regain optimal use but the end result is often some degree of post-traumatic stiffness. As with Volkmann contracture, function can sometimes be improved with surgery to enhance motion of the damaged structure or with a surgical procedure to transfer a normal structure to the injured area.

Complex Regional Pain Syndrome

One poorly understood cause of post-traumatic contracture is a process called *complex regional pain syndrome* (CRPS). Persons with CRPS report hypersensitivity or a burning sensation, skin color and hair growth changes, and alterations in normal sweat patterns. Typically, the disease is confined to one extremity and usually follows trauma or surgery. The exact cause, however, is unknown.

Physicians speculate that CRPS is related to damage or dysregulation in the nervous system. Most cases of CRPS are termed type I (reflex sympathetic dystrophy), with no history of focal nerve injury. CRPS type II (causalgia) refers to persons with a confirmed history of nerve damage. In both types of CRPS, the nerves to the arm lose their ability to properly control blood flow, sensation, and temperature. As a result, the extremity becomes swollen, painful, excessively warm or cool, and stiff. Permanent contractures follow as tendons and ligaments become scarred.

A *syndrome* is defined by identifiable *symptoms* (what the patient experiences) and *signs* (what the health care professional finds) as opposed to any formal diagnostic studies. Nonetheless, *thermography* (skin temperature testing) and a bone scan to check for abnormal bone metabolism can reveal abnormalities early. Nerve conduction studies can reveal nerve compression, as in carpal tunnel syndrome. X-rays can show osteoporosis of the involved limb.

Treatment of complex regional pain syndrome. Treatment for CRPS is directed at ameliorating pain and preserving function. Early intervention is best; at whatever stage treatment begins, prolonged treatment may be needed to deal with the effects of chronic pain. The *American Idol* judge and singer Paula Abdul recently revealed that she struggled for years with CRPS related to an injury that occurred when she was a teenager. Earlier diagnosis and treatment would have most likely helped resolve her pain much sooner.

Most treatments for CRPS are nonsurgical. Patients participate in regularly scheduled therapies to reduce swelling and increase mobilization of tendons and joints. Biofeedback methods are often used to help the person gain control over hypersensitivity and temperature changes. Dysfunctional nerves in the neck can be temporarily "turned off" with a series of injections known as *ganglion blocks*. Narcotic medicines will limit the pain, too, but should be used carefully and for a short period only to avoid long-term dependence. Steroids are useful, early, to decrease swelling. In the long term, *neuroactive medicines* (drugs used for seizures or depression) have become the drugs of choice for symptom management. Surgery is rarely necessary and is reserved for cases of ongoing peripheral nerve dysfunction, such as carpal tunnel syndrome or a painful nerve stump (*neuroma*).

CONGENITAL PROBLEMS

Cerebral Palsy

Cerebral palsy (CP) is a term that encompasses a host of static brain disorders that cause motion problems as well as disorders of cognition, communication, and other neurologic functions. Most cases of CP are attributed to disturbances in the brain during fetal development, but the exact nature of those disturbances is not understood. A small number of cases result from damage to the brain at birth or in the first several years after birth.

Worldwide, the incidence of cerebral palsy is about 2 out of every 1,000 live births—regardless of location, race, or socioeconomic status. Premature babies are more likely to have CP. Advances in medicine have not appreciably changed the prevalence of cerebral palsy or solved the mystery of the in utero dysfunction that causes it. Although these cerebral injuries are not progressive, they are also not curable.

Most persons affected by CP develop spasticity. The problem is usually apparent by 6 to 9 months of age, as children with CP typically have difficulties sitting and standing. It is less common for the upper limbs to be affected but when they are, a host of challenges—to personal hygiene, feeding, and other activities of daily living—present themselves. The first indication of spasticity in the hand can be failure to achieve tip-to-tip pinch between the thumb and index finger by 1 year of age. In addition, the arm is characteristically held in flexion at the elbow with the hand turned down, the wrist flexed, and the thumb in the palm. The child's fingers may be flexed or extended.

Nonsurgical treatment for cerebral palsy affecting the hand. Occupational therapy for the hand affected by cerebral palsy begins at an early age, with efforts to stretch spastic muscles, strengthen antagonistic weak muscles, and minimize contractures. Splints and other orthotics are used as adjuncts to the regular exercises overseen by the child's parents and therapists. Most often, these devices are worn at night so as not to interfere with daytime activities. The spectrum of muscular dysfunction varies from no voluntary control to full voluntary hand use. Hence, the goals of therapy and, ultimately, surgery, can range from improved ability to manage personal hygiene to restoration of a specific function of the hand or wrist.

Many persons with CP have normal intelligence but it is masked by difficulties speaking and writing. Christopher Nolan, a noted Irish poet and author who was born in 1965, suffered a lack of oxygen during birth that caused his cerebral palsy. Nolan could move only his head and eyes yet he attended college and eventually, with the use of a pointer attached to his forehead, wrote an award-winning book of international acclaim, *Under the Eye of the Clock* (his autobiography). The standup comedian Josh Blue is giving audiences a greater appreciation for the struggles of those with cerebral palsy. His jokes arise from his experiences living with CP and in 2006 earned him the Last Comic Standing award on NBC's reality show. He coined the term *palsy punch* as a smart way to fight, explaining it this way: "First of all, they don't know where the punch is coming from, and second of all, neither do I."

Surgical treatment for cerebral palsy affecting the hand. Surgery for the upper limb in a person who has cerebral palsy should be considered with great care. When an affected person has already adapted fairly well and become accustomed to her contractures, it's important to remember that surgical interventions may leave the extremity weak and useless. Similarly, a well-intentioned wrist procedure may make finger function worse if the "big picture" of the patient's integrated upper extremity function is not considered. The best surgical plan can only be based on careful observation of the person, a thorough understanding of her disability, and solid experience treating the spastic hand. When surgery is determined to be a good option, it is often performed just before the child reaches school age.

Functional gains after surgery are usually only seen in those with some previous baseline voluntary use of the hand. A person who has greater disability will generally gain improved hygiene and appearance, both of which enhance quality of life. Surgery to correct contracture in a child's hand typically involves adjusting soft tissue to release or transfer tight muscle tendon units. Wrist flexor tendons, for example, may be moved to the top of the hand to gain wrist extension or to the fingers to achieve finger extension. Excessively tight finger or thumb flexor tendons can be lengthened to open up the hand. Ultimately, some contractures do become fixed. Adolescent or adult patients often benefit from a wrist fusion to put the hand in a more functional position, combined with soft tissue surgery to improve the function of the fingers.

Arthrogryposis Multiplex Congenita

Fixed contractures are a part of a congenital disorder known as *arthrogryposis multiplex congenita*. Arthrogryposis is a non-progressive disease occurring in 1 out of every 3,000 live births. It is thought to be caused by decreased fetal movement. Motion may be limited by fetal abnormalities in the muscle, nerve, or connective tissue. Alternatively, motion may be restricted by maternal abnormalities related to the uterine environment, infections, drug use, or other causes. It is believed that up to 30 percent of cases may have a genetic cause. Joint contractures develop with weakness and fibrosis of the associated muscles.

Typically, all of the person's extremities are affected by the disease. People with severe arthrogryposis have central nervous system, eating, and respiratory difficulties. The upper extremity usually rests with the shoulder rotated inward, the elbow extended, the palm down, and the wrist and fingers flexed—a highly dysfunctional position. Although vigorous therapy and splinting can help stretch contractures, surgical release is often necessary to improve function. As with people who have cerebral palsy, in people who have arthrogryposis, the entire function of arm and hand needs to be considered before operating on any one part. Most children with arthrogryposis have normal intellect and language development, and go on to lead successful lives as adults. Celestine Harrington, a person with arthrogryposis and quadriplegia and author of the 1996 book, *Some Crawl and Never Walk*, is one such person.

Treatment for arthrogryposis. Generally, surgery on the arm is delayed until after the child has entered school, usually at about age 5 or 6. At the most basic level, one arm should be able to be used for eating (flexed elbow) and the other for toileting (extended elbow). Both of these activities rely on a shoulder with some internal rotation. As children with arthrogryposis adapt to their contractures, the surgeon must be careful not to remove what has become a functionally advantageous deformity. For example, rotating the humerus (arm bone) outward may appear more normal but will make it difficult for the child to feed herself. Similarly, a child with an extended elbow may become dependent on an extreme wrist flexion contracture to eat, so the deformity should not be taken away.

Surgical procedures include joint releases (*capsulotomies*) and muscle releases or transfers to improve power. The elbow extension contracture can be released, allowing elbow flexion that's powered by sliding the forearm muscles above the elbow or transferring the triceps or pectoralis across the elbow. If the elbow can be successfully mobilized, a wrist flexion deformity may be addressed next. Mildly contracted wrists can be straightened by removing a row of wrist bones; more severe contractures require fusion of these bones. The fingers and thumb are then opened by releasing or lengthening the attached tendons and sometimes fusing the knuckle joints.

STROKE AND TRAUMATIC BRAIN INJURY

Our control of our arms and hands is a result of electrical signals sent from our brains. When the brain is damaged, motor nerves are disrupted and there is loss of voluntary (deliberate) motion. A *stroke* (sometimes called a *brain attack*) is caused by an interruption of blood supply to the brain, while trauma directly affects the brain in a mechanical fashion. Whatever the origin of the damage to the brain, affected limbs usually become spastic and contracted. The acute problems of stroke and traumatic brain injury are different, however.

Strokes tend to occur in older persons when a blood vessel in the brain becomes clogged with a clot or ruptures. Symptoms develop suddenly and are determined by the part of the brain that has been damaged. Most strokes affect the motor center in the brain that controls the arms, speech, and facial motion for one side of the body. Other symptoms include an acute change in mental status, difficulty communicating, headache, and loss of coordination. Strokes are medical emergencies and can cause permanent neurologic damage and death. Immediate medical attention is required. If you can get medical care, preferably at a designated primary stroke center, within 3 hours of the onset of symptoms, the stroke can usually be stopped and the effects reversed.

For the first 24 to 48 hours after a stroke that is not addressed or not treated in time, flaccid paralysis is common. Then, increased muscle tone gradually becomes noticeable over the course of days or weeks. In the upper arm and hand, spasticity becomes apparent in the shoulder and eventually migrates down the arm. There is a characteristic inward rotation of the shoulder along with flexion of the elbow, wrist, and fingers. Spasticity will subside as voluntary motor control improves. Spontaneous neurologic recovery usually peaks at about 6 months after a stroke. People who have significant spasticity should undergo intensive therapy and splinting during this period of potential neurologic recovery.

Traumatic brain injuries typically occur in younger persons as a result of a car crash, a fall from a great height, a sports injury, or other blunt trauma to the head. Most people involved in trauma also suffer from associated orthopedic and organ damage, and these issues are usually at the forefront of the concerns of the emergency room doctor caring for the patient. Spasticity and rigidity will become apparent within days, prompting splinting and range of motion therapy. Traumatic injury can also cause extra bone, known as *herterotopic ossification*, to form around joints, further limiting motion.

The long-term prognosis after traumatic brain injury is most dependent on the person's age. Children and young adults demonstrate the most potential for neurologic recovery. As with stroke patients, motor control may plateau by about 6 months. In some cases, however, neurologic function improves for up to 18 months, prompting the frequent use of injectable and oral medications as a temporary way to control muscle spasticity. For example, young patients with strong muscles benefit from Botox injections (temporarily paralyzing the muscles) combined with casting or splinting to stretch muscles. These interventions may also be used in stroke patients with particularly severe spasticity.

Treatment for Stroke and Traumatic Brain Injury

Upper extremity surgery for stroke or traumatic injury is considered only when neurologic function has reached a steady state. The patient must be able, cognitively, to participate in his postoperative care and therapy in order to reach realistic goals after surgery. Surgery may be as simple as removing heterotopic bone to mobilize an elbow in an otherwise normal extremity. Or it may be as straightforward as cutting the tendons to the hand and wrist to allow better hygiene in an extremity with no voluntary muscle control. More complex surgeries to lengthen or transfer tendons and correct deformities can be undertaken in persons who have muscle imbalances and the ability to follow basic instructions.

BURN CONTRACTURES

Burns to the hand and upper extremity can be caused by flames of a fire or by exposure to excessive heat, cold, electricity, or chemicals. Whatever the cause, the injury can lead to a common denominator— contracture. During the evaluation and treatment of all burns, the hand must be considered a high priority. In fact, the best way to treat burn contractures is to prevent or minimize them though aggressive early burn management.

Thermal Burns

Thermal burns are classified based on depth. *Superficial or partial thickness burns* result in redness and blistering, while *full thickness burns* leave white "leathery" skin. Most partial thickness burns heal spontaneously with conservative measures such as antibiotic creams and exercises focused on maintaining mobility.

Areas of full thickness burns will not regrow skin and must be treated with surgical debridement and skin grafting. Particularly deep circumferential burns can cause excessive pressures similar to the compartment syndrome described earlier in this chapter. *Escharotomy* is the surgical process of cutting the tight, leathery tissue to release the pressure. Splinting always plays a critical role, keeping the hand in a functional position during the time that it remains swollen and painful to move. Splints will limit the claw position the hand commonly adopts after severe trauma.

Treatment for thermal burn contractures. Even with the best burn management, contractures can still occur. The thumb is prone to falling into the palm while the fingers tend to contract (extended at the knuckles and flexed at the smaller joints). Often, the scar can be surgically excised, affected joints and tendons can be mobilized, and a skin graft can be placed on the wound bed. Tight bands of scar tissue, such as those pulling the thumb into the palm, can be lengthened by plastic surgery techniques such as *Z-plasty*. In difficult cases, the hand may need to be resurfaced with more viable tissue from another area of the body. Tissue transfer involves lifting skin and subcutaneous tissue from another area (often the leg) and transferring it along with an attached blood supply to the hand.

Electrical Burns

Electrical burns cause readily apparent thermal-like injury to the skin, but concealed deep tissue damage is a notorious problem. Burns from low-voltage (less than 1,000 volts) exposure are managed much like thermal burns. Areas of full thickness damage are removed and grafted while early therapy and splinting maintain a reasonable hand position and function. Burns from direct contact with high voltage (greater than 1,000 volts) results in extensive death to the deep tissues, including muscles, blood vessels, nerves, and bones.

Treatment for electrical burns. Damage from an electrical burn will require multiple surgeries to repeatedly assess the wound and remove dead tissue. Tight muscle compartments are released the way they would be with any compartment syndrome. If little viable tissue remains after sequential surgeries, amputation may be the last best option. Otherwise, surgical reconstruction begins, using healthy tissues from other parts of the body.

Chemical Burns

Chemicals cause skin and soft tissue burns much like thermal or low-voltage electrical injuries. But unlike those exposures, chemicals typically remain in contact with the skin, causing progressive tissue damage. Sometimes there is little initial pain, such as with exposure to lime in ordinary wet cement. Other burns, such as those from hydrochloric acid in pool cleaners, are readily apparent.

Treatment for chemical burns. The critical step in treatment of a chemical burn is early dilution or neutralization of the chemical substance. Most chemicals can be adequately diluted with 1 to 2 hours of a water lavage or immersion soaking. In other cases, special agents may be needed. For example, cleaning agents containing phenol may need to be removed from the skin with glycerol. Likewise, ongoing ulcerations from hydrofluoric acid–based rust removers may be best stopped by injections of calcium gluconate. Splinting and therapy are essential parts of treatment and, ultimately, contractures that develop are treated as any others caused by burn mechanisms—dead or scarred tissue is removed and replaced with a skin graft or tissue transfer from another part of the body.

◆

At first glance, contracture and spasticity can affect one's hand function much like the many other disorders discussed in this book. But on a fundamental level, the contracted or spastic hand is limited in more than recreational and work activities. The form, the cosmetic appearance of this hand, limits the hand's effectiveness as a vehicle for emotional expression and communication. That is why the treatment strategies discussed in this chapter should not be considered for function only. An improvement to a hand afflicted by contracture or spasticity opens a portal to the outside world.

CHAPTER 11

WHERE DO WE GO
FROM HERE?

♦

Future Innovations in Hand Surgery

James P. Higgins, M.D.

Hand surgery as a subspecialty is relatively young. Specialized training in hand surgery in the United States didn't even begin until after World War II, unlike its parent subspecialties—plastic surgery, orthopedic surgery, general surgery, and neurosurgery—some of which go back centuries. Despite its relatively short history, however, hand surgery has seen explosive change and rapid progress in the treatment of injuries and diseases that affect the hand. What the future holds for such a dynamic specialty is impossible to predict. As always, looking ahead requires understanding the past. Examining the events and challenges that have stimulated innovation in hand surgery so far provides insights that will give us a glimpse into the future of this surgical specialty.

The three areas that form the building blocks for the future of hand surgery and that demonstrate the most marked innovations are microsurgical reconstruction of the hand, upper extremity prosthetics, and hand allotransplantation.

MICROSURGICAL RECONSTRUCTION
OF THE TRAUMATIZED HAND

No single development has had as profound an impact on the field of hand surgery as the advent of microsurgical techniques. The ability to repair nerves and blood vessels smaller than what the unaided eye can see heralded an accelerated phase of discovery and innovation that hand surgery continues to harness. Microsurgery has redefined which diseases and injuries are correctable and has made previously unimaginable stories of recovery commonplace.

The term *microsurgery* was first coined in 1960 to describe the experimental success of two surgeons, Drs. Julius Jacobson and Ernesto Suarez, in repairing 1 to 2 millimeter blood vessels in a dog (used as a model for trials of the technique) in Burlington, Vermont. Before this, vascular surgeons were capable of repairing arteries of larger sizes with the use of the same crude magnification used by jewelers or seamstresses—magnifying glasses of +2 power.

Drs. Jacobson and Suarez employed a microscope designed for surgery on the inner ear. This level of magnification enabled the surgeons to repair vessels comparable in diameter to angel hair pasta with enough accuracy to establish and maintain blood flow across the microscopic repair site. Since that time, the subspecialty of microsurgery has become much more precise, advanced, and routine.

Before 1960, a number of factors laid the foundation for the birth of microsurgery. The original technique of connecting (*coapting*, or *anastomosing*) two blood vessels was first performed by Dr. Alexis Carrel in 1902, for which he won the Nobel Prize in 1912. This suturing technique, although now modified with better instrumentation, is in part still the basis of how blood vessels are connected today. Additionally, the development of the microscopes in the 1920s for use in ear and eye surgery provided a prototype for microsurgical microscopes. Although microsurgical technique today is applied to many subspecialties— including head and neck surgery, obstetrics and gynecology, urology, and neurosurgery—the period of rapid expansion that began in the 1960s was born primarily of the needs and innovations of the developing subspecialty of hand surgery.

The origins of microsurgery cannot be adequately recounted without describing the profound contributions of Dr. Harry Buncke, who has been called "the father of microsurgery." The idea of using microsurgical techniques for arm and hand surgery was conceived by Dr. Buncke while working with his colleague, Dr. Tom Gibson, in Glasgow, Scotland, in 1957. After returning to his home in San Francisco, without any applicable equipment or materials, Dr. Buncke set up a microsurgical workshop in his garage. There, he set about creating sutures small enough to be used to repair 1 millimeter diameter blood vessels (the size of a large grain of sand).

At the time, commercially available suture material was far too large. Dr. Buncke created and developed his own microsuture by metalizing individually separated threads of silk from silkworm fiber. He obtained one of the first three operating microscopes developed by Dr. Jules Jacobsen and modified it for the purposes of microsurgery. He adapted jewelers' instruments and began his experimentation. First, Bunke focused on small blood vessels in the ears of rabbits, with the goal of transecting (cutting) the blood vessel, repairing it, and maintaining blood supply to the ear. It was not until his fifty-seventh attempt that he succeeded, a testimony to his persistence, dedication, and optimism.

The next 10 years saw a series of new applications of microsurgery to treat the traumatized hand. At that point in history traumatic loss of digits, hands, and arms was treated solely by closure of the amputated stump. The ability to perform microsurgical *anastomosis* (connection) of blood vessels opened the door for what was termed *replantation*, the reattachment of amputated parts. Surgeons already had the ability to repair bone, skin, and muscle injuries. Replantation was never thought possible, however, because of one critical remaining gap: reestablishment of blood flow to the amputated part. With the ability to repair blood vessels of 1 or 2 millimeter diameter, traumatic amputations could now be considered repairable.

In 1962, Drs. Ronald Malt and Charles McKhann performed the first replantation (reattachment) of a completely severed arm on a 12-year-old boy in Boston, and in 1963, Dr. Zhong-Wei Chen and colleagues performed the first successful replantation of an amputated hand in

Shanghai, China. The first replantation of an individual digit (a severed thumb) was achieved by Drs. Shigeo Komatsu and Susumu Tamai in Japan in 1968. Successful reattachment of amputated arms, hands, and digits showed the incredible achievements microsurgery could bring. The seemingly impossible was now possible.

The ensuing decades saw the continued expansion of microsurgical techniques to further improve upper extremity reconstruction. Once microsurgeons were able to replant a severed part, they began to employ the same skills to move tissue from one part of the body to another to replace missing parts when replantation was not possible (such as in crush injuries or burns). This radical concept was first applied to finger reconstruction. In search of a mechanically and functionally similar substitute for amputated fingers, reconstructive surgeons sought to use toes for finger replacement. In 1966, Dr. Chen and his team in Shanghai used the second toe as a transferred part to replace missing fingers. This technique of harvesting uninjured parts from elsewhere in the body to reconstruct injured areas was termed *free tissue transfer* and the parts were referred to as *free flaps*. In an effort to more closely approximate the size, strength, and function of the thumb, in 1967, Dr. John Cobbett, a colleague of Dr. Buncke, performed the first great toe transfer to re-place an amputated thumb. The surgery was a success; the transplanted "thumb" survived and was useful to the patient.

The concept was taken a step further during the 1970s when, al-most simultaneously, teams from the United States, Australia, and Japan began to harvest other flaps of tissue, including skin, fat, muscle, and bone, to be moved from one part of the body to an area in need. Success of the transfer relied on successful anastomosis and subsequent blood supply to the transferred part.

Reconstructive surgery truly flourished with the successful use of microsurgical technique. Unlike *transplantation*, where organs are har-vested from donors and require lifelong use of medications to limit the patients' immune response to a "foreign" tissue, free tissue transfer re-quires no such medical management. The patient is both the donor and the recipient.

As the concept of free tissue transfer was used for an increasingly wider range of problems, reconstructive microsurgeons began to take inventory of all of the tissues in the body that could be safely and reliably harvested for use elsewhere. Many of the early innovations in this field, and particularly the innovations that are currently ongoing, were in hand surgery. Today the concept and technique of free tissue transfer has been incorporated into the treatment not only of trauma but also for cancer reconstruction, infection treatment, burn management, and congenital deformities of all parts of the human body.

Although the initial advances in microsurgery were centered on the reestablishment of blood flow through small blood vessels, upper extremity trauma also benefited: now nerve injuries could be treated, too. With use of the operating room microscope (figure 11.1), surgeons were better able to assess the extent of nerve damage from trauma and apply the developing principles of nerve repair to restore critical function and sensation to the injured hand. Pioneers in this field began to harvest uninjured nerves from other parts of the body to reconstruct deficits in the arm with nerve grafting. Nerve grafting makes it possible to replace damaged nerves with undamaged tissue; the cost is removal of functional nerves from other parts of the body, often resulting in areas of poor or absent sensation elsewhere, a problem that led to the development of synthetic nerve graft substitutes or conduits in the form of tubes made of absorbable materials. These tubes have yielded promising results for microsurgical nerve repair and are currently the subject of intense research and scientific testing.

Advances in *microvascular* (blood vessel) and *microneural* (nerve) reconstruction have been very rapid and have served as the foundation for contemporary hand surgeons' overall progress in treating the hand. Although microsurgery has helped surgeons achieve what was previously unimaginable, we are still in a very dynamic phase and, I believe, greater achievements are still to come.

In the world of microvascular hand surgery, we are now traveling toward new accomplishments in another medical frontier. We have achieved reattachment (replantation) of amputated parts; replacement of amputated parts with similar parts (as in toe transfers); and grafting of tissue from elsewhere in the body onto blood vessels. With these successes to encourage us, we are entering a phase where the inventory of donor sites will become nearly limitless. As surgeons strive to

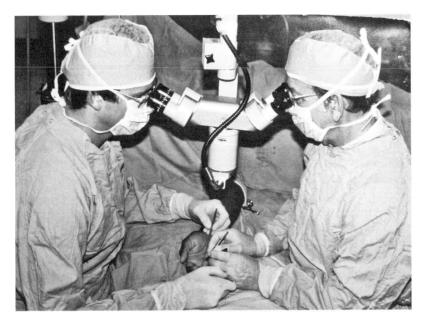

Figure 11.1. Dr. Raymond M. Curtis (right) at the operating microscope. COURTESY THE
CURTIS NATIONAL HAND CENTER

anastomose progressively smaller blood vessels, teams from around the
globe are describing previously unidentified flaps from nearly all tissue
territories, essentially making the entire body a source for potential
tissue transfer—all to the incredible benefit of the patient.

A second major development in this technology is in the use of pre-
fabricated and prelaminated flaps, terms coined in the 1990s. In *prefabrication*, surgeons insert a blood vessel into tissue that is thought to be
ideal for harvest. Once the blood vessel has provided adequate blood
flow to the desired tissues, the surgeons can harvest the tissue on the
implanted blood vessel. Perfection of this technique further allows surgeons to harvest the ideal tissue, enabling them to create a source vessel
of adequate size, length, and caliber for whatever need the patient has.

In *prelamination*, surgeons create complex three-dimensional structures that require different tissue (such as bone, cartilage, and fat) with
one or more preliminary surgical procedures before moving it as a composite flap in a final operation. An example is the use of cartilage or
bone that is "buried" underneath skin or fat in an area where a flap can

readily and easily be harvested after the inserted tissues have developed blood supply from the surrounding subcutaneous tissue.

Both of these techniques (prefabrication and prelamination) further expand the hand surgeon's ability to harvest exactly what the patient needs from a portion of the body that can most readily provide it.

The third area of microvascular surgery that may further improve hand surgery techniques is the development of blood vessel substitutes. Traditionally, blood vessels have been replaced with grafts of veins harvested from elsewhere in the body. The development of synthetic vessel substitutes, particularly experimental models made from collagen, shows promise. The conduits (*synthetic vessel substitutes*) perform well and the person's own cells replace the inner lining of the conduit, thereby making it a more normal blood vessel.

NERVE RECONSTRUCTION

The field of microsurgery will not only accelerate hand surgery through microvascular techniques but also through microneural techniques. The field of peripheral nerve reconstruction for upper extremity injuries is extremely dynamic. Synthetic nerve conduits are now fairly widely used, but the extent of their usefulness is still undefined. Many surgeons and scientists are focusing their efforts on other ways of accelerating nerve injury recovery, including the use of immunosuppressive medications. It is still unclear if these methods will prove to be superior to synthetic nerve conduits or more conventional nerve grafting.

Following a different line of research, some surgeons are attempting to accelerate nerve root growth by performing procedures called *nerve transfers*. This technique uses the uninjured functioning nerves found in the same area as the nearby injured nerves for coapting (connecting) neural regenerative fibers close to their target point. In the case of sensory nerves, the coaptation would occur as close as possible to the target tissue of skin that the nerve must innervate. In this way, a "live wire" can be brought as close to the area of reconstruction as possible, minimizing the time for recovery and maximizing its likelihood. All of these efforts are moving forward independently while benefiting from shared discoveries and ideas. Time will demonstrate which of these innovations carries microsurgery of the hand and arm into the next era of advancement.

UPPER EXTREMITY PROSTHETICS

While the world of microsurgery focused on reconstructing the traumatized upper extremity, the field of prosthetics was seeing rapid advances in the development of synthetic replacements of the upper extremity.

In patients with amputations at various levels of the upper extremity, three conventional prosthetic options have evolved. The first are *cosmetic silicone prostheses*, which are most typically used for replacement of amputated fingers. These prosthetics are molded and cast of silicone, and artistically rendered to be the shape, size, color, and appearance of the person's fingers. Artists are employed to paint the inside of the prostheses to provide an exact match to an individual's skin tone and provide the visual appearance of texture and even surface features such as hair. (Painting is done on the inside of the prosthesis so that normal use does not mar the finish.) Although these prostheses provide a very satisfying cosmetic result, they do not give the person the ability to control motion of the finger, to feel the finger, or to use the finger in a highly functional manner.

The second type is a *body-powered cable prosthesis*, generally used for amputations at the upper arm level. These are harnessed to the person's remaining extremity and have a cable rigging akin to bicycle cables. Movement of the shoulder manipulates the cables to open and close the hand replacement device. Although these prostheses are functionally superior to the cosmetic prostheses, only one joint can be manipulated at a time, making it cumbersome to use and limiting its function. The person using a body-powered cable prosthesis needs to manually position the elbow and wrist in space with the opposite hand and use the shoulder harness to open and close the hand itself.

The third option is a *myoelectric prosthesis* (figure 11.2). These prostheses harness the body's ability to contract muscles in the amputation stump. The small electrical impulses transmitted by the contraction of the muscles are detected by surface skin–level electrodes, much like an EKG (electrocardiogram) detects contractions of the heart. These surface electrodes are placed on the inner socket of the myoelectric prosthesis and their signal is amplified, enabling the prosthetic hand to

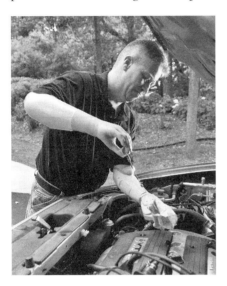

open and close. In this way, the person can learn to flex certain muscle groups to open the hand and others to close the hand. Although this invention is a great stride forward, only one joint can be activated at a time. It also requires a significant amount of training for the person to learn to flex the specific muscle groups that make the opening and closing of the prosthetic more natural. These limitations result in a prosthetic that requires the wearer to spend a great deal of time on routine activities of daily life.

Figure 11.2. Myoelectric prosthesis.
COURTESY OTTOBOCK

The field of prosthetic development has recently undergone a surge of innovation, primarily due to the needs of military casualties. Recent military conflicts, particularly in the Middle East, have generated devastating extremity injuries due to roadside bombs and IEDs (improvised explosive devices). In previous conflicts, many of the injured would not have survived but, now, because of better body armor, transportation, and medical care in the immediate area, even the severely injured are surviving. As a result, there has been an increase in research funding and interest in the development of both upper and lower extremity prosthetics that provide a greater degree of function, quicker and more effective rehabilitation, and a higher level of proficiency with routine tasks.

Most of these injuries occur in young adults, and their need for functional extremities (whether a prosthetic or a full transplant) is paramount. For the young adult who has lost multiple limbs, the importance is heightened. Imagine the individual who has lost both hands;

what a stunning improvement to his life to get back one of them or, better yet, both.

In 2001, a team headed by Dr. Gregory Dumanian in Chicago performed the first of a series of landmark procedures for upper arm amputees. The first patient was a 54-year-old, bilateral shoulder-level amputee as the result of a devastating electrical injury. The team employed a new technique called *targeted muscle reinnervation* (TMR). Their goals were to create a myoelectric prosthesis that could operate multiple joints simultaneously and would require less training for the user to achieve proficiency. Their plan was to use the transected (cut) nerves in the amputation stump that had previously controlled the hand and to connect these nerves to shoulder, upper arm, and chest wall muscles. In this way these muscles could amplify the brain signals that were originally transmitted through the nerves to control the hand.

Previous prosthetics, including conventional myoelectric prosthetics, had harnessed contractions of the muscles in the amputation stump to create movement in the prosthetic hand. These muscles were not initially intended for hand function, however, and use of these prosthetics required significant retraining on the part of the patient. By harnessing the function of previously non-utilized amputated nerves in the amputation stump, Dr. Dumanian's team hoped that patients could ultimately use the same nerve pathways they had learned since birth to operate the routine functions of the hand. The median nerve, used for flexing the fingers, could be transferred to a chest wall muscle. After months of healing, when the nerve grew into the chest wall muscle, the man noticed a twitching there when he focused his thoughts on flexing his fingers. The electrodes from the targeted muscle reinnervation prosthesis were situated above the muscle and sent impulses to flex the hand.

Likewise, other nerves to the upper extremity (radial nerve, ulnar nerve, musculocutaneous nerve), with each of their inherent tasks, were transferred to separate and distinct muscles in the chest wall, shoulder girdle, and upper arm. When the patient focused on opening his fingers, one portion of the shoulder might twitch; when he focused on rotating his palm downward, a portion of the upper arm might twitch. With electrodes placed on targeted muscles, multiple joints could be motorized in the prosthesis, requiring very little training. To activate this function with the prosthesis, all the patient had to do was think about performing the function, just as he had before amputation. This remarkable concept met with great success. Since the initial patient, other hopeful amputees have undergone similar and progressively more complex procedures and achieved continually improved functional outcomes.

On standard tests, individuals treated with targeted muscle reinnervation demonstrated as much as a 250 percent increase in their overall upper extremity function. This level of function was previously thought to be unobtainable. It has always been thought that prosthetic replacement of amputated parts could never equal that of replantation because prosthetics don't offer sensation. Even a prosthesis with the greatest functional motor recovery would never be used as much as a normal hand or arm because there isn't sensory feedback regarding temperature, texture, firmness, and so forth, of the objects being grasped.

Remarkably, Dr. Gregory Dumanian of Chicago and his team have taken this concept a step further to address this deficit of sensation. For the most recent patients undergoing targeted muscle reinnervation, the surgeons are using *targeted sensory reinnervation* (TSR). In this procedure, not only are motor nerves controlling rerouted motor function, but the nerves that initially provided sensation to the person's hand are providing sensation. These sensory nerves are rerouted and coapted to nerves that provide sensation to the skin of the upper chest wall and shoulder. The operation was initially performed on a 24-year-old woman who had sustained an amputation in 2004. In 2005, she underwent a combination of targeted motor reinnervation and targeted sensory reinnervation and has, thus far, experienced great success. Her prosthesis has a grid of 128 electrodes on the surface of the skin. Some of these are used to detect muscle twitches to enable her to open and close her hand and control her elbow. She has noted detectible sensation in 20 selected areas on her upper chest wall and shoulder. When these areas are touched, the woman feels sensation that she interprets as tips of her fingers, the palm of her hand, and so forth. After mapping out these areas of her skin, the team hopes to develop a more state-of-the-art prosthesis that will send signals to the electrodes from her hand that indicate the temperature and texture of objects the prosthesis touches or grasps. In the past decade, prosthetic development has seen an incredible acceleration in its innovation, which has set the stage for an exciting and promising future for upper extremity amputees.

HAND TRANSPLANTATION

While the world of prosthetics was advancing in its ability to restore function via artificial means, and microsurgery was advancing surgeons' capabilities in replanting amputated parts or replacing parts with tissue from elsewhere in the body, a third dimension of upper extremity reconstruction was being explored: hand transplantation. The field of composite tissue allotransplantation has emerged, making the ability to replace amputated and injured hands with donor hands a reality.

Donor-organ transplantation had its roots in World War II. Drs. Peter Medewar and Thomas Gibson experimented with donor skin grafting to treat injured servicemen in Scotland. For this work, Dr. Medewar received a Nobel Prize, as well as knighthood. In 1954, the plastic surgeon Dr. Joseph Murray led a team in Boston to perform the first successful solid organ transplant—a kidney donated from one identical twin to the other. Four years later, he performed the same procedure on fraternal twins and won the Nobel Prize for this work. Dr. Murray opened the field of solid organ transplantation, which is common today.

In order to undergo organ transplantation, the patient's immune system needs to be suppressed, or it will reject the donated part. Initially, bone marrow was radiated for this purpose, and the patient took immunosuppressive drugs. As medications improved, the success of kidney, liver, heart, pancreas, and other organ transplantation became more reliable. Regardless of improvements, the medications exposed patients to serious side effects and long-term risks, including an increased chance of infection, the development of drug-induced diabetes, increased incidence of the development of cancers, and diminished wound healing. Although this profile of medication side effects would normally be considered quite severe, the risks were deemed acceptable given the life-threatening conditions—kidney failure, liver failure, heart failure—that were being treated.

The use of transplantation for reconstruction of the hand was considered unlikely because, although functionally devastating, the loss of an upper extremity is not life-threatening. For this reason, the potential adverse side effects of immunocompromising medications would for many decades outweigh the benefits of transplantation of hands and arms.

An additional hurdle in the development of hand transplantation was the immunogenicity of skin. Unlike a solid organ, the hand is composed of several different types of tissue: bone, muscle, tendon, fat, and skin. The success of hand transplantation would require controlling the immune response and potential for rejection of all of these. The skin is the tissue most apt to create an immune response and result in rejection. The pursuit of transplantation of such a body part was termed *composite tissue allotransplantation* (CTA) and later also referred to as *vascularized composite allotransplantation* (VCA). Surgeons around the country who focused on the prospects of transplantation of hands to replace amputated and injured parts were joined by specialists from other fields who were pursuing replacement of damaged composite tissue structures (face, larynx, and abdominal wall transplantation) to improve a person's function after a traumatic injury.

The origins of composite tissue allotransplantation can be traced back to Dr. Earle Peacock, a plastic surgeon from North Carolina. Dr. Peacock was a pioneer in his pursuit of CTA principles in the reconstruction of the upper extremity. His work focused on replacing the tendons that flex the fingers, as well as the complex ligament-derived pulley system that enables this complex and intricate system to achieve *prehension*, knowing where your hand is in space. After his initial procedure in 1957, more than 40 such reconstructions were performed by a small number of surgeons using tendon and pulley mechanisms from unmatched cadavers. These surgeries were performed without any immunosuppressive medications, and the technique was an improvement on the previously unsolved problem of flexor tendon scarring and injury. This landmark development, however, was overshadowed by the attention being paid to the development of solid organ transplantation during this same era. Also, Dr. Peacock's flexor tendon sheath reconstructions were eclipsed by the development of implantable silicone tendon replacement rods. Nonetheless, early composite tissue allotransplantation provided hand surgeons with advanced techniques to restore function. In 1960, an attempt at the first hand transplantation (performed in Ecuador by Dr. Robert Gilbert) failed due to acute rejection 3 weeks after the procedure. Multiple pioneers failed in their attempts at transplanting extremities in experimental animal models, and the field of composite tissue allotransplantation was temporarily abandoned. It was believed that the immunogenicity of skin was too great a hurdle to overcome.

As more effective and less toxic immunosuppressants—like Imuran in the 1960s, cyclosporin in the 1980s, and tacrolimus in the 1990s—were used in solid organ transplantation, the stage was set for a revival of composite tissue transplantation. The most dramatic step forward occurred in the mid-1990s when one of the newest agents, mycophenolic acid (MMF), used in combination with tacrolimus during a limb transplantation experiment on an animal model, was successful. The door was opened for clinical trials in humans.

With only partial support from the larger field of hand surgery, scientists in selected centers around the world proceeded with human trials. The first modern-day allotransplantation of the hand was performed in September 1998 in Lyon, France, by a team headed by Dr. Jean-Michel Dubernard. Their success was rapidly followed by the first American hand transplantation in January 1999 by a team headed by Dr. Warren Breidenbach in Louisville, Kentucky. Many incredible "firsts" followed, leading up to January 2000, when the first bilateral hand transplantation was performed in Lyon. In 2012, a combined team of surgeons from Johns Hopkins Hospital (led by Drs. W. P. Andrew Lee, Gerald Brandacher, and Jaimie Shores) and the surgeons of The Curtis National Hand Center (including myself and many of the contributors to this book) performed the most complex and extensive bilateral arm transplantation to date. The surgical technique and medical treatment of hand transplant patients continues to evolve each year.

Various other composite tissue allotransplantation models have been pursued. A team of surgeons led by Dr. Guenter Hoffman moved forward with composite tissue transplantation of human knees. Dr. Marshall Strome became a pioneer as his team in Cleveland, Ohio, performed groundbreaking work in composite tissue allotransplantation of the human larynx. Facial transplantation for patients sustaining massive deforming and debilitating facial injuries was also pioneered by Dr. Dubernard's team in France when he performed a facial transplant in November 2005. The second such facial transplantation was performed in China by Dr. Guo and his team in April 2006.

As each of these areas of CTA progressed, the general public and the surgeons in the respective specialty fields become more accepting of the functional and aesthetic outcomes, as well as the risks of the immunosuppressive medications. Now it appears that composite tissue allotransplantation is a clinical reality and it will, no doubt, escort in an explosive era of innovation and progress in the treatment of upper extremity issues.

Three critical successes seem to ensure the role of composite tissue allotransplantation in the future of hand surgery. The first is successful control of the immunogenic response to allotransplantation of skin, as mentioned earlier. The second is the increasingly improved medication regimens to control the patient's immune response and risk of rejection. The amount and number of medications required are being reduced and side effects are decreasing. The goal of continued experimental efforts in this field is to achieve what was previously unthinkable: immuno-tolerance without medications. Many researchers firmly believe that such an achievement is not only feasible but is something we will see in the near future. With the severe side effects of the immunosuppres-sion medications erased, more widespread acceptance and use of trans-plantation technology will be developed. The third factor that seems to promise a long and bright future for the use of CTA technology in the upper extremity is the unanticipated observation that the regeneration of sensory and motor nerves in the transplanted parts has exceeded that of standard nerve repair and hand replantation. One of the side effects of some of the immune-compromising medications, particularly tacrolimus, is acceleration of nerve regeneration and regrowth. Many conventional hand surgeons have for years been skeptical of CTA be-cause of poor functional returns due to inadequate nerve regeneration. It appears, however, that researchers have made breakthroughs that are leading to good functional and sensory outcomes.

By the end of 2013, more than 60 patients around the globe had received either unilateral or bilateral hand/arm transplantation. Other composite tissue allotransplantations as well have been performed in many more patients. It appears that within the past decade the concept of composite tissue allotransplantation—born from the efforts of pioneers of the 1950s—has undergone a phase of rapid growth and widespread acceptance.

HISTORY OF HAND SURGERY

Hand surgery was born of a need to address a changing medical landscape. Dr. Asa Sterling Bunnell, the physician credited as the founding father of hand surgery, served in the U.S. military in France during World War I (figure 11.3). His exposure during the war to undertreated upper extremity wounds sparked a lifelong passionate interest in care of the hand and a legacy from which everyone in this field has benefited. Between the World Wars, Dr. Bunnell studied, practiced, and wrote extensively on the surgical treatment of the hand. He published what, at the time, was recognized as the foremost authoritative textbook on the subject and defined the subspecialty in a manner that was considered radical. He believed that adequate treatment of the hand required a surgeon who could accomplish all the tasks normally performed by

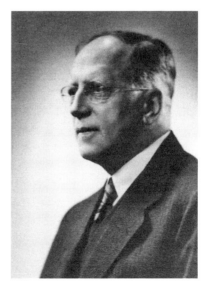

Figure 11.3. Dr. Asa Sterling Bunnell, the physician credited as the "founding father" of hand surgery. COURTESY THE CURTIS NATIONAL HAND CENTER

several different subspecialists. The hand surgeon would need to be skilled in the treatment of nerve, bone, muscle, tendon, blood vessel, and skin disorders and wounds as they relate to the entire upper extremity. This unusual combination of necessary skills created the specialty of hand surgery.

In 1943, Franklin Delano Roosevelt appointed the first orthopedic surgeon ever to be elevated to the position of surgeon general of the army. His selection of Dr. Norman T. Kirk was speculated by some to be due in part to Roosevelt's particular appreciation and understanding of the importance of orthopedic surgery and rehabilitation given his affliction and struggle with polio since the age of 39.

Dr. Kirk was a longtime friend, colleague, and admirer of Dr. Bunnell. Charged with the massive task of overseeing the care of the wartime wounded, Kirk immediately requested that Dr. Bunnell serve as a civilian consultant to the Army Medical Corps to head the "crippled hand" service. Dr. Bunnell accepted and, at age 62, closed his busy practice in San Francisco and started nine centers for hand surgery at medical hospitals around the country. He selected young leaders to direct these centers, and personally toured each one, giving lectures, performing surgeries, and training the future leaders in hand surgery. From the nine centers, eight of the directors went on to become presidents of the specialty's premier academic association, the American Society of Surgery of the Hand, and today all are still considered leaders in the specialty of hand surgery.

Before Dr. Bunnell's appointment to the Army Medical Corps, war injuries involving the hand were universally viewed to be so profoundly and permanently debilitating that treatment was neglected or assigned to the least experienced surgeons. Dr. Bunnell's and Dr. Kirk's writings describe their astonishment at the frequent and indiscriminate use of amputation for wartime hand injuries.

If surgeons during World War II were asked to speculate about the future of hand surgery, they would likely not have predicted the progress that has occurred in such a short time. They would probably be surprised by the number of academic centers and medical units dedicated to the advancement of treatment of the hand. The span and scope of research, clinical advancements, instrumentation, procedures, and rehabilitation programs for disorders of the hand has been so great during the past 60 years as to be nearly unimaginable. The stories of reconstruction and recovery of hands from injuries previously thought untreatable are today truly astonishing.

Now, in an era of highly specialized and advanced techniques in hand surgery, with decades of contributions from general surgeons, orthopedic surgeons, plastic surgeons, neurosurgeons, therapists, and prosthetists, it may seem that we have reached a point after which we will see no further improvement. With the advantage of experience and history, we are certain that this will not be the case. It is difficult to provide a comprehensive inventory of all of the subfields and areas of scientific inquiry that continue to drive hand surgery forward; fracture fixation, joint replacement, imaging, joint mechanics, tumor management, and arthritis management—all are continually improving.

I believe, however, that our field is currently experiencing the most rapid growth in areas focused on the reconstruction of the injured hand. When my colleagues and I began work on this book, the acceleration in these fields was due in part to U.S. wartime engagements. In our professional societies and national meetings, it is clear that treatment of wartime trauma is becoming the more common point of discussion and an area of innovative treatment.

◆

While the entire field of hand surgery has enjoyed a dynamic history from its relatively recent formative years on, it appears that it is going through an accelerated phase that promises to herald an era of improved technologies, improved procedures, and, most important, improvement in the care of those people stricken with injuries or disease of the upper extremity. While these advances are happening foremost in the areas of microsurgery, prosthetics, and transplantation, a multitude of other advances are occurring in a wide variety of subfields of hand surgery. We look forward with great anticipation to continued innovation and progress in our field.

RESOURCES

◆

American Association for Hand Surgery
www.handsurgery.org

American College of Rheumatology
www.rheumatology.org

American Diabetes Association
www.diabetes.org

American Foundation for the Blind
www.afb.org

American Sign Language/ National Association for the Deaf
http://www.nad.org/issues/american -sign-language

American Society for Reconstructive Microsurgery
www.microsurg.org/patients/awareness/

American Society for Surgery of the Hand
www.assh.org

Centers for Disease Control and Prevention
www.cdc.gov/diabetes and www.cdc.gov /arthritis

Helping Hands Foundation: Connecting families of children with upper limb loss
www.helpinghandsgroup.org/

Jim Abbott Foundation
www.jimabbott.net/

Limb Differences: An online resource for families and friends of children with limb differences
limbdifferences.org/

National Institute on Deafness and Other Communication Disorders (NIDCD)
www.nidcd.nih.gov

National Institute of Arthritis and Musculoskeletal and Skin Diseases
www.niams.nih.gov

Stop Sports Injuries
www.stopsportsinjuries.org

The Arthritis Foundation
www.arthritis.org
www.arthritistoday.org

The Braille Institute
www.brailleinstitute.org

The Curtis National Hand Center
www.curtishand.com

CONTRIBUTORS

◆

W. Hugh Baugher, M.D., Clinical Faculty, The Curtis National Hand Center, MedStar Union Memorial Hospital, Baltimore, Maryland.

Kevin C. Chung, M.D., 1994–1995 Curtis National Hand Fellow, Section of Plastic Surgery, Department of Surgery, Professor of Orthopaedic Surgery, University of Michigan Medical School, Ann Arbor, Michigan.

Philip Clapham, B.S., Department of Surgery, The University of Michigan Health System, Ann Arbor, Michigan.

Christopher L. Forthman, M.D., Clinical Faculty, The Curtis National Hand Center, MedStar Union Memorial Hospital, Baltimore, Maryland.

Thomas J. Graham, M.D., Former Chief of The Curtis National Hand Center, Chief Innovation Officer, Cleveland Clinic Innovations, Cleveland, Ohio.

James P. Higgins, M.D., Chief of Hand Surgery, Clinical Faculty, The Curtis National Hand Center, MedStar Union Memorial Hospital, Baltimore, Maryland.

Ryan D. Katz, M.D., Clinical Faculty, The Curtis National Hand Center, MedStar Union Memorial Hospital, Baltimore, Maryland.

Michael A. McClinton, M.D., Clinical Faculty, The Curtis National Hand Center, MedStar Union Memorial Hospital, Baltimore, Maryland.

Kenneth R. Means Jr., M.D., Clinical Faculty, Clinical Director of Research, The Curtis National Hand Center, MedStar Union Memorial Hospital, Baltimore, Maryland.

Rebecca J. Saunders, P.T., Certified Hand Therapist, The Curtis National Hand Center, MedStar Union Memorial Hospital, Baltimore, Maryland.

Keith A. Segalman, M.D., Clinical Faculty, The Curtis National Hand Center, MedStar Union Memorial Hospital, Baltimore, Maryland.

E. F. Shaw Wilgis, M.D., Emeritus Chief, The Curtis National Hand Center, MedStar Union Memorial Hospital, Baltimore, Maryland.

Raymond A. Wittstadt, M.D., Clinical Faculty, The Curtis National Hand Center, MedStar Union Memorial Hospital, Baltimore, Maryland.

Neal B. Zimmerman, M.D., Clinical Faculty, The Curtis National Hand Center, MedStar Union Memorial Hospital, Baltimore, Maryland.

Ryan M. Zimmerman, M.D., 2014-2015 Curtis National Hand Fellow, The Curtis National Hand Center, MedStar Union Memorial Hospital, Baltimore, Maryland.

INDEX

◆